# My Supermarket Sidekick

## Your Aisle-by-Aisle Shopping Guide

Bonnie R. Giller, MS, RDN, CDN, CDE

The information in this book is for informational and educational purposes only. It is not intended as a substitute for professional medical advice or the care of a physician. Do not use this information to diagnose or treat a health problem or disease. If you suspect you have a health problem, please contact your health care provider.

To my husband, Michael, for always believing in me and cheering me on to achieve my goals and dreams.

To my children, Matthew and Shaina, Jason, Jennifer and Lauren for your love of healthy food and for being proud to be the children of a registered dietitian nutritionist.

To my grandson, Evan, who puts a smile on my face ALWAYS!

To my newborn grandson, Zach, I can't wait for you to taste grandma's food!

To my parents, Ruth and Danny Berger. There are no words to express how grateful I am for all you have taught me and for being my guiding light in life and in business. Thank you, thank you, thank you!

To my clients, who give me the inspiration to continue creating new products and services. Your nutrition questions and thirst for knowledge gives me the motivation to keep on doing what I love. Thank you.

And, last but not least, thank you to my assistant Samantha Baturin. Samantha had a creative vision for this book and took that vision and made it a reality. Many thanks for all the hours you spent formatting, designing and taking photographs for the book. You are one of a kind!

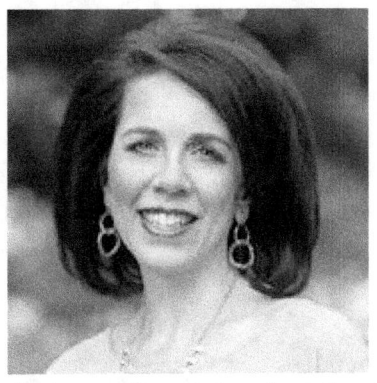

## About the Author

Bonnie R. Giller helps people struggling to lose weight and people with medical conditions like diabetes and irritable bowel syndrome take back control so they can get the healthy body and life they want. She does this by creating a tailored solution that combines three essential ingredients: a healthy mindset, caring support and nutrition education. The result is they lose weight, keep it off, and avoid medical complications so they can live a healthy life symptom free.

Bonnie is a Registered Dietitian Nutritionist (RDN), Certified Dietitian-Nutritionist (CDN), Certified Diabetes Educator (CDE) and a Certified Intuitive Eating Counselor. She offers programs for the chronic dieter to achieve long lasting weight loss, for people with diabetes to attain blood sugar control and prevent diabetes complications, and for those suffering with irritable bowel syndrome to identify their food triggers so they can enjoy a symptom free life. Bonnie also treats a variety of other medical conditions, and provides nutrition presentations and Lunch and Learn seminars to the community and local organizations.

Bonnie is very passionate about helping her clients regain the trust in themselves and their bodies so they can live the life they are meant to live.

Get your free copy of Bonnie's e-book **5 Steps to a Body You Love Without Dieting** and learn more about intuitive eating at DietFreeRadiantMe.com.

For more information about Medical Nutrition Therapy to treat diabetes, IBS and other medical conditions, visit BRGHealth.com.

# Table of Contents

Introduction                                                    1

Know Before You Go: Tips for Your Shopping Trip                 3

Navigating the Label                                            5

Food Labeling Terms                                             7

Fruits & Vegetables                                            11

Vegetarian Proteins                                            17

Deli Meats                                                     21

Meat & Poultry                                                 25

Fish & Seafood                                                 31

Dairy: Milk, Yogurt, Cheese, & Dairy Alternatives             37

Eggs                                                           43

Grains                                                         47

Hot & Cold Cereal                                             53

Dry & Canned Foods                                            57

Sauces & Condiments                                           63

Snacks                                                        69

Frozen Foods                                                  75

Beverages                                                     81

References                                                    83

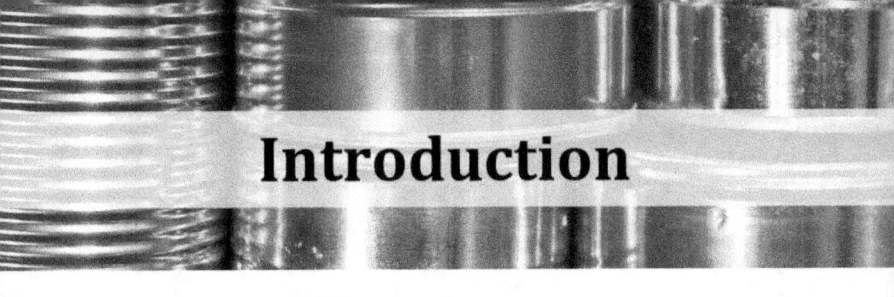

# Introduction

In today's day in age there is a growing concern about choosing the right foods to reach and maintain a desirable weight and good health. You probably think you are picking out nutritious wholesome foods when you go food shopping, however, the wording and slogans on food packages can be deceiving. Manufacturers often want you to believe a food is healthy for you, yet unfortunately they are not telling you the whole story.

I wrote **My Supermarket Sidekick** as a guide to prepare you before you go food shopping, explain what to look for when reading nutrition labels and ingredients lists while you are shopping, and to help you navigate through the food aisles when at the supermarket. I included additional nutrition tips and guidelines to help you successfully choose only the best products for optimal health and wellness.

**My Supermarket Sidekick** is a quick and easy pocket guide to help you reach your health goals. I am confident that this guide will act as just that- your Sidekick when food shopping, your best friend and partner in your food trip excursion. Carry it in your bag or pocket while at the store and flip through it aisle-by-aisle for quick and easy answers to all your nutrition questions while grocery shopping.

In good health,
Bonnie

# Know Before You Go

## *Tips for Your Shopping Trip*

1. Keep an ongoing shopping list on the refrigerator or in another convenient spot each week. When you finish an item in the house, add it to the list.

2. Plan meals ahead so you know what ingredients you will need for the week.

3. Variety and moderation are key to achieving and maintaining a healthy lifestyle. Try to buy one new fruit, vegetable, or grain each week to expand your family's tastes.

4. Do a big food shopping trip once a week. This will make it less likely for you to impulse buy when making quick stops at the grocery store.

5. Separate your shopping list into the aisles similar to the way they are listed in My Supermarket Sidekick to stay organized and focused.

6. Check the newspaper and circulars for coupons. Only pull out coupons that are a normal part of your daily shopping list.

7. Do not go to the supermarket on an empty stomach! You are more likely to stray away from foods on your list, and will buy more than is needed.

8. Don't give in to unhealthy foods your children may want. It's ok to say no!

# Know Before You Go

## *Tips for Your Shopping Trip*

9. Shop around the perimeter of the store for the freshest products that are the least processed.

10. Compare labels when buying food items. Ingredients and nutrients vary between brands.

11. Look for items with shorter ingredient lists that include ingredients you can read and recognize.

12. Be aware of serving size. The information listed on the nutrition label will indicate nutrients per serving, not for the whole package.

# Navigating the Label

**Serving Size**
Indicates serving size and how many servings are in the package. The nutrition facts listed will reflect the amount for a single serving size which may not be the same as the amount you choose to eat.

**% Daily Value**
The percent daily value is based on a 2000-calorie diet. These percentages show how a single serving compares to the daily value for the entire day.

**5% or less** is considered low. Generally aim for low total fat, saturated fat, trans fat, cholesterol, and sodium.

**Calories from Fat**
This indicates how many calories of the total calories are from fat.

**Protein**
Notice the DV for protein is not included. This is because most individuals consume more than the DV.

## Nutrition Facts

Serving Size 1 cup (110g)
Servings Per Container About 6

**Amount Per Serving**

**Calories** 250  Calories from Fat 30

| | % Daily Value* |
|---|---|
| **Total Fat** 7g | **11%** |
| Saturated Fat 3g | **16%** |
| *Trans* Fat 0g | |
| **Cholesterol** 4mg | **2%** |
| **Sodium** 300mg | **13%** |
| **Total Carbohydrate** 30g | **10%** |
| Dietary Fiber 3g | **14%** |
| Sugars 2g | |
| **Protein** 5g | |

| | |
|---|---|
| Vitamin A | 7% |
| Vitamin C | 15% |
| Calcium | 20% |
| Iron | 32% |

* Percent Daily Values are based on a 2,000 calorie diet. Your daily value may be higher or lower depending on your calorie needs.

| | Calories: | 2,000 | 2,500 |
|---|---|---|---|
| Total Fat | Less than | 55g | 75g |
| Saturated Fat | Less than | 10g | 12g |
| Cholesterol | Less than | 1,500mg | 1,700mg |
| Total Carbohydrate | | 250mg | 300mg |
| Dietary Fiber | | 22mg | 31mg |

**Carbohydrates**
The three types of carbs are sugars, fiber, and starches. At least 50% of your total daily carb intake should be from whole grains.

**Sugars**
Notice there is no percent DV for sugar. It is advised to limit sugar consumption.

# Food Labeling Terms

**Calories**

❖ <u>Calorie Free</u>: less than 5 calories per serving.

❖ <u>Low Calorie</u>: 40 calories or less per serving.

❖ <u>Reduced or Fewer calories</u>: At least 25% less calories than the original version.

**Fat**

❖ <u>Saturated Fat Free</u>: Less than 0.5 grams saturated fat per serving and less than 1% of total fat from trans fat.

❖ <u>Low Saturated Fat</u>: 1 gram or less saturated fat per serving and no more than 15% of calories from saturated fat.

❖ <u>Fat Free</u>: Less than 0.5 grams fat per serving and does not contain ingredients that are fats.

❖ <u>Low Fat</u>: 3 grams or less fat per serving.

❖ <u>Reduced or Less Fat</u>: at least 25% less fat than the original version.

**Cholesterol**

❖ <u>Cholesterol Free</u>: Less than 2 milligrams of cholesterol and 2 grams or less of saturated fat per serving.

❖ <u>Low Cholesterol</u>: 20 milligrams or less cholesterol and 2 grams or less saturated fat per serving.

❖ <u>Reduced or Less cholesterol</u>: At least 25% less cholesterol per serving than the original version and 2 grams or less of saturated fat per serving.

# Food Labeling Terms

**Sodium**

❖ <u>Salt Free, Sodium Free, Unsalted</u>: Less than 5 milligrams sodium per serving and does not contain sodium chloride (table salt).

❖ <u>Very Low Sodium</u>: 35 milligrams or less sodium per serving.

❖ <u>Low Sodium</u>: 140 milligrams or less sodium per serving.

❖ <u>Reduced or Less Sodium</u>: At least 25% less sodium per serving than original version.

**Other**

❖ <u>Fortified or Enriched</u>: Vitamins and/or minerals added to a product in amounts at least 10% above levels that are present in food.

❖ <u>Fortified</u>: Used when nutrients were not originally present in food.

❖ <u>Enriched</u>: Means nutrients were lost in processing and added back in.

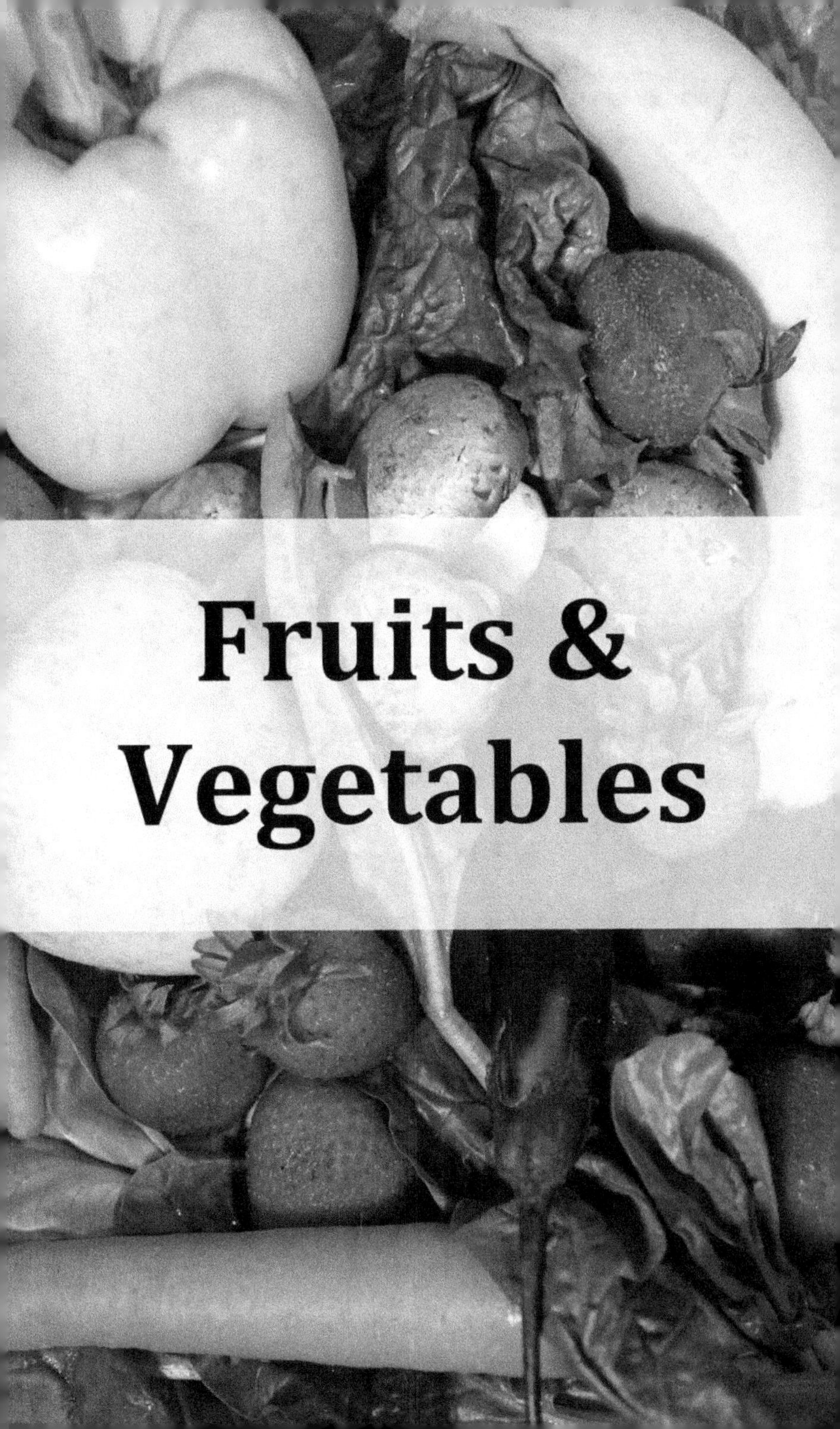

# Fruits & Vegetables

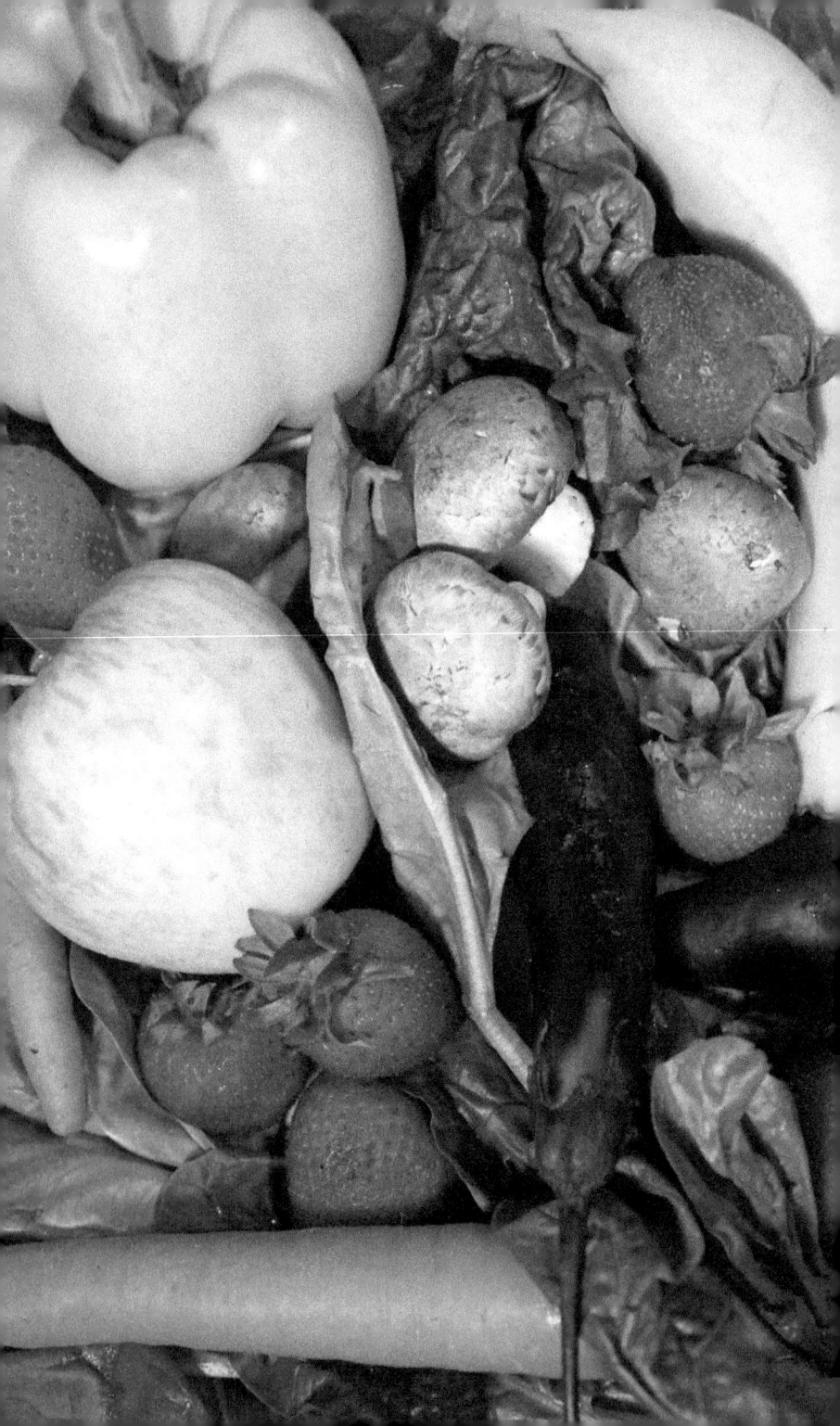

# Fruits & Vegetables
## *Navigating the Label*

❖ Packaged produce may display a Nutrition Facts Label. If not, check for a poster or pamphlet for nutrition information or ask the store manager to provide this information.

❖ Fruits are naturally low in fat with the exception of avocado and coconut.

❖ Whole fruits and vegetables are a source of dietary fiber, helping you feel full.

❖ Most vegetables are low in sugar with exceptions such as beets, carrots, corn, peas, potatoes, and winter squashes.

❖ Fruits naturally contain more sugar than vegetables. The sugars found in fruit are "simple" sugars which are easily digested by the body.

❖ Organic produce mean the plants were grown with the use of natural pesticides rather than synthetic pesticides.

❖ Non-organic produce may have been treated with chemical herbicides and pesticides.

*See the chart on the next page to learn more about which produce typically are exposed to heavy pesticide use, thus are recommended to buy organic, and which tend to be grown with less pesticides.*

# Fruits & Vegetables

## Navigating the Label

### The Dirty Dozen+

*These produce are highly exposed to pesticides and are best to choose organic options.*

| | | |
|---|---|---|
| Apples | Nectarines | Strawberries |
| Celery | Peaches | Sweet Bell Peppers |
| Cherries | Potatoes | +Hot Peppers |
| Cucumbers | Snap Peas | +Kale |
| Grapes | Spinach | +Collard Greens |

### The Clean Fifteen

*These produce have less exposure to pesticides and are fine to buy non-organic.*

| | | |
|---|---|---|
| Asparagus | Eggplant | Papaya |
| Avocado | Grapefruit | Pineapple |
| Cabbage | Kiwis | Sweet Corn |
| Cantaloupe | Mangoes | Sweet Potatoes |
| Cauliflower | Onions | Sweet Peas (frozen) |

*Reference: ewg.org*

# Fruits & Vegetables

## *Shopping Tips*

❖ Choose a variety of colors and types of fruits and vegetables for greater profile of nutrients. Think of a rainbow when filling your cart, different colors all offer different nutrients!

❖ Shop seasonally when possible to get fresh produce that contain more nutrients and flavor at a lower cost.

❖ Only choose ripe produce when they will be eaten right away. If you are not going to be consuming a fruit or vegetable for a few days, it is best to choose the almost ripe pieces.

❖ Keep produce that have a longer shelf life in stock at home such as apples, citrus fruits, carrots, broccoli, potatoes and Brussel sprouts.

❖ Fresh fruits and vegetables may be found pre-sliced or pre-chopped for when you don't have time to prep or if you're not comfortable handling a knife.

❖ Freeze your own fruits and vegetables when they are on sale or if you cannot finish them when they are ripe. Wash and fully dry produce and then put in freezer bags. Layering parchment paper throughout the bag will reduce clumping.

❖ Dried fruit has a long shelf life but can be high in sugar and calories. Look for options with no sugar added.

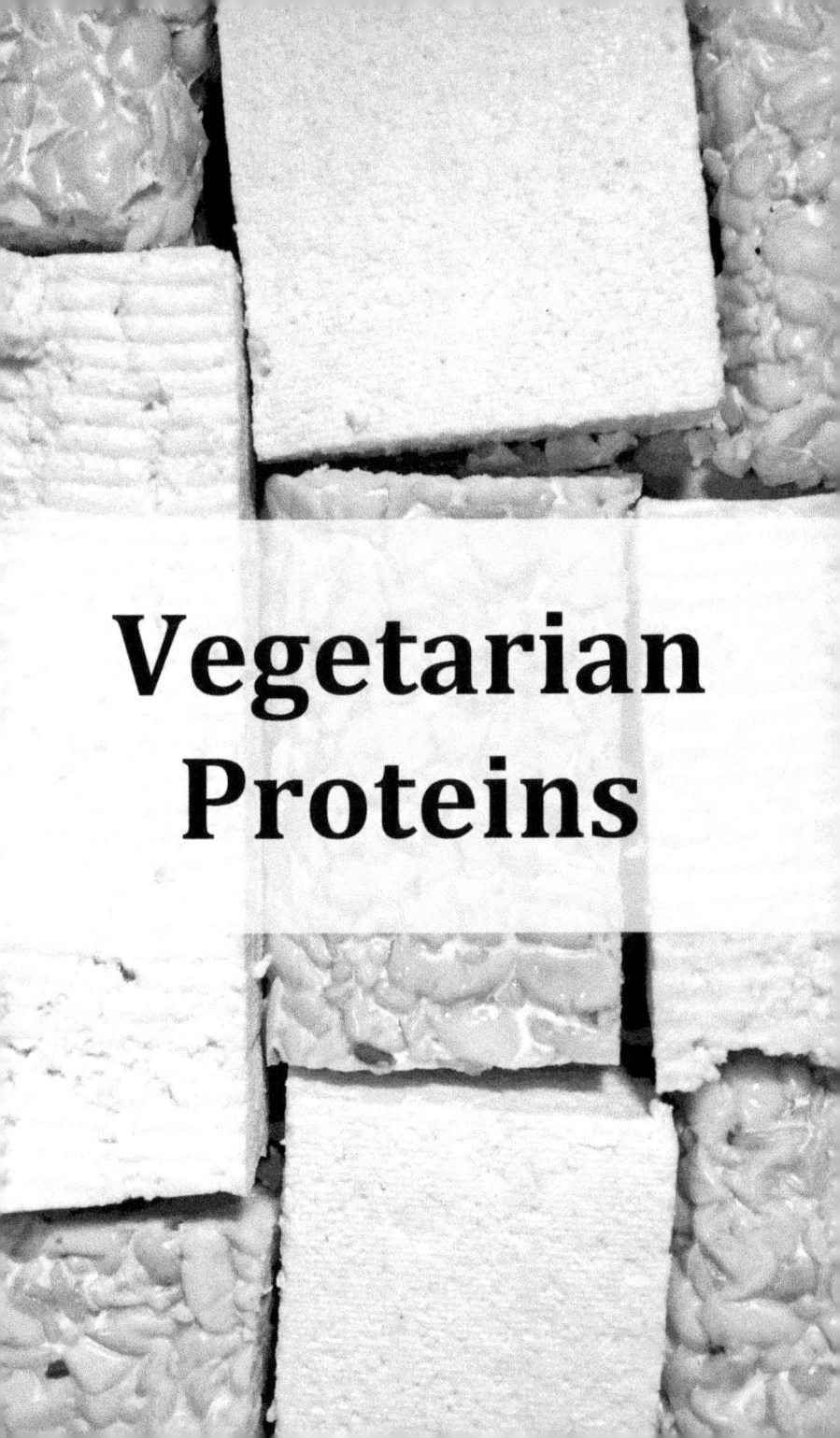

# Vegetarian Proteins

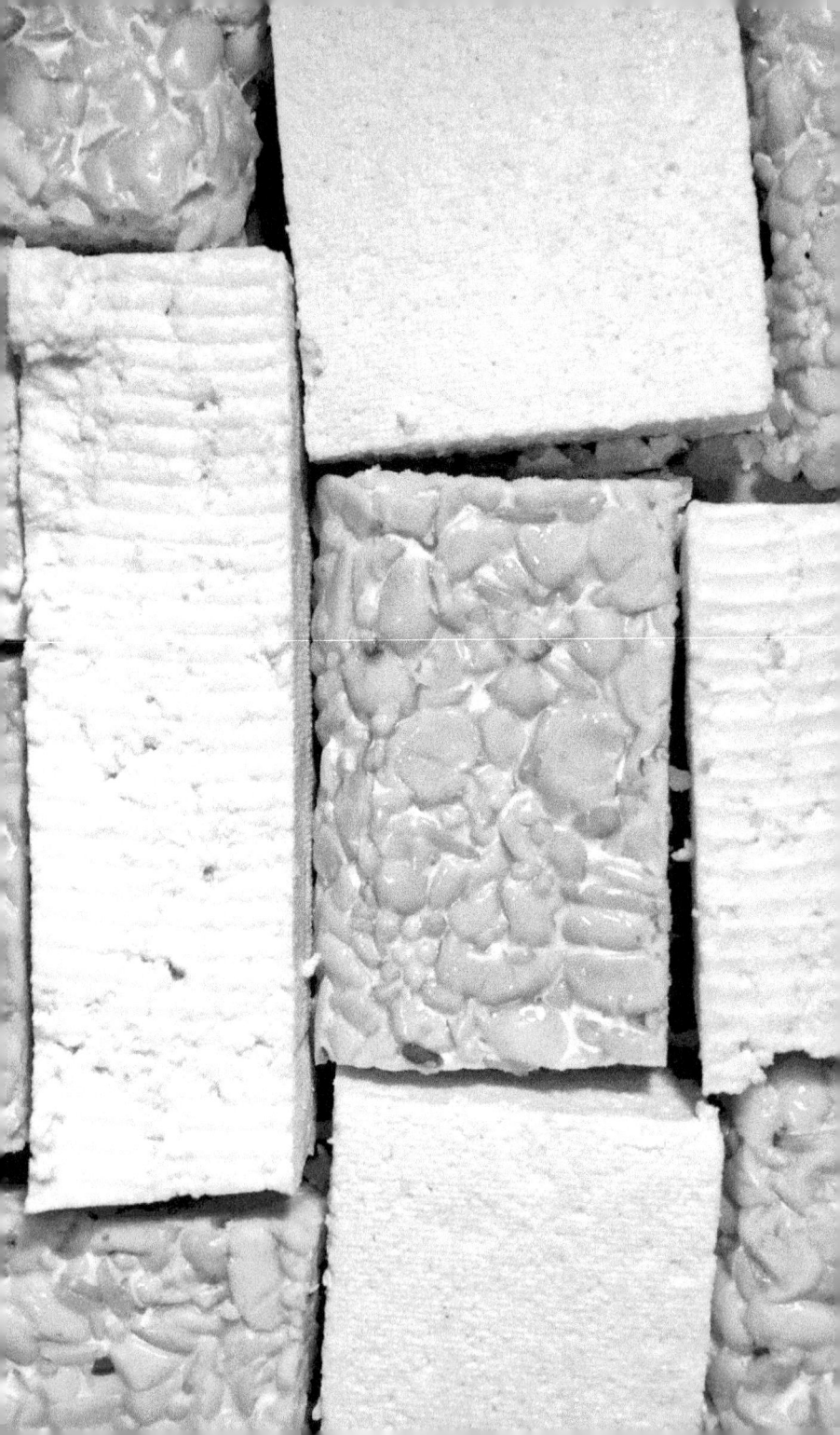

# Vegetarian Proteins

## *Navigating the Label*

❖ **Tofu or Bean Curd**
›  Made from curdled soymilk pressed into blocks.
›  ½ cup serving: ~10 grams protein.
›  **Silken Tofu**: Very soft texture, ideal for blending, making creamy sauces, or use in creamy desserts.
›  **Firm or Extra Firm Tofu**: Ideal for baking, grilling, or sautéing. It is recommended to follow directions for draining liquids and then to marinade for at least 30 minutes before cooking.

❖ **Tempeh**
›  Made from fermented soybeans and grains. This is denser and has a grainy texture compared to tofu. It is recommended to marinade for at least an hour before cooking.
›  ½ cup serving: ~15 grams protein.
›  Ideal for baking or grilling.

❖ **Seitan**
›  Made from wheat gluten.
›  3 ounce serving: ~20 grams protein.
›  Typically used to imitate meat.

❖ **Edamame**
›  Immature soybeans, usually boiled or steamed in the pod.
›  ½ cup serving: ~8 grams protein.
›  A high-quality, complete source of protein.

# Vegetarian Proteins

## *Shopping Tips*

❖ It is possible to get adequate protein on a plant-based diet. Be sure to eat a variety of these foods each day to achieve your protein goals.

❖ Always remember to check the labels on premade imitation meats and veggie burgers. Some are prepared with sauces and additives that increase calorie, sodium, and fat content.

❖ Follow the instructions for preparation on tofu, tempeh, and seitan. Most packages offer recommendations on how long the product should be marinated before cooking for optimal flavor.

❖ For more plant-based protein options, head over to the <u>Canned and Dry Foods</u> aisle. Beans, nuts, and seeds are great sources of protein.

  › 1 cup soy beans: 29 grams protein.

  › 1 cup garbanzo beans: 11 grams protein.

  › 1 ounce almonds: 6 grams protein.

  › 1 ounce flax or chia seeds: 5 grams protein.

❖ Soybeans and soy protein foods are a plant-based source of protein that are low in saturated fat and cholesterol.

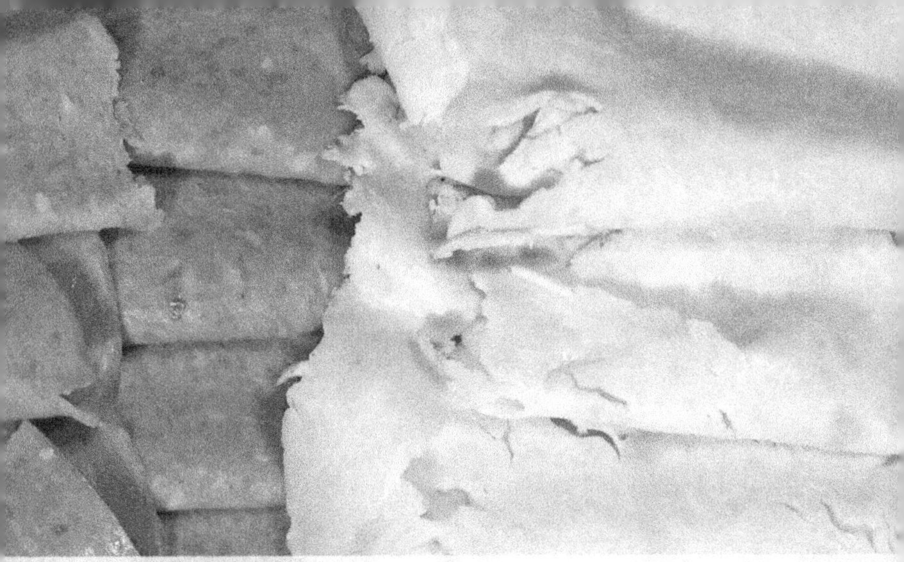

# Deli Meats

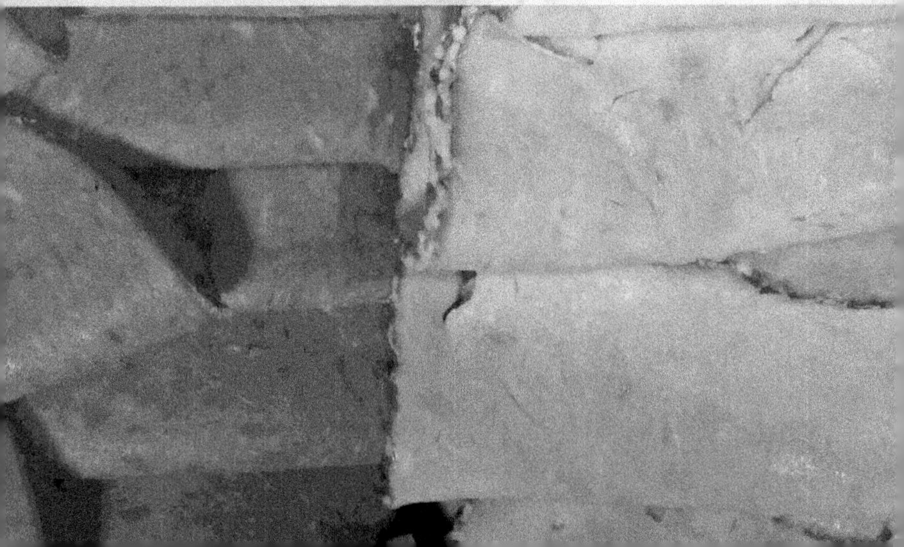

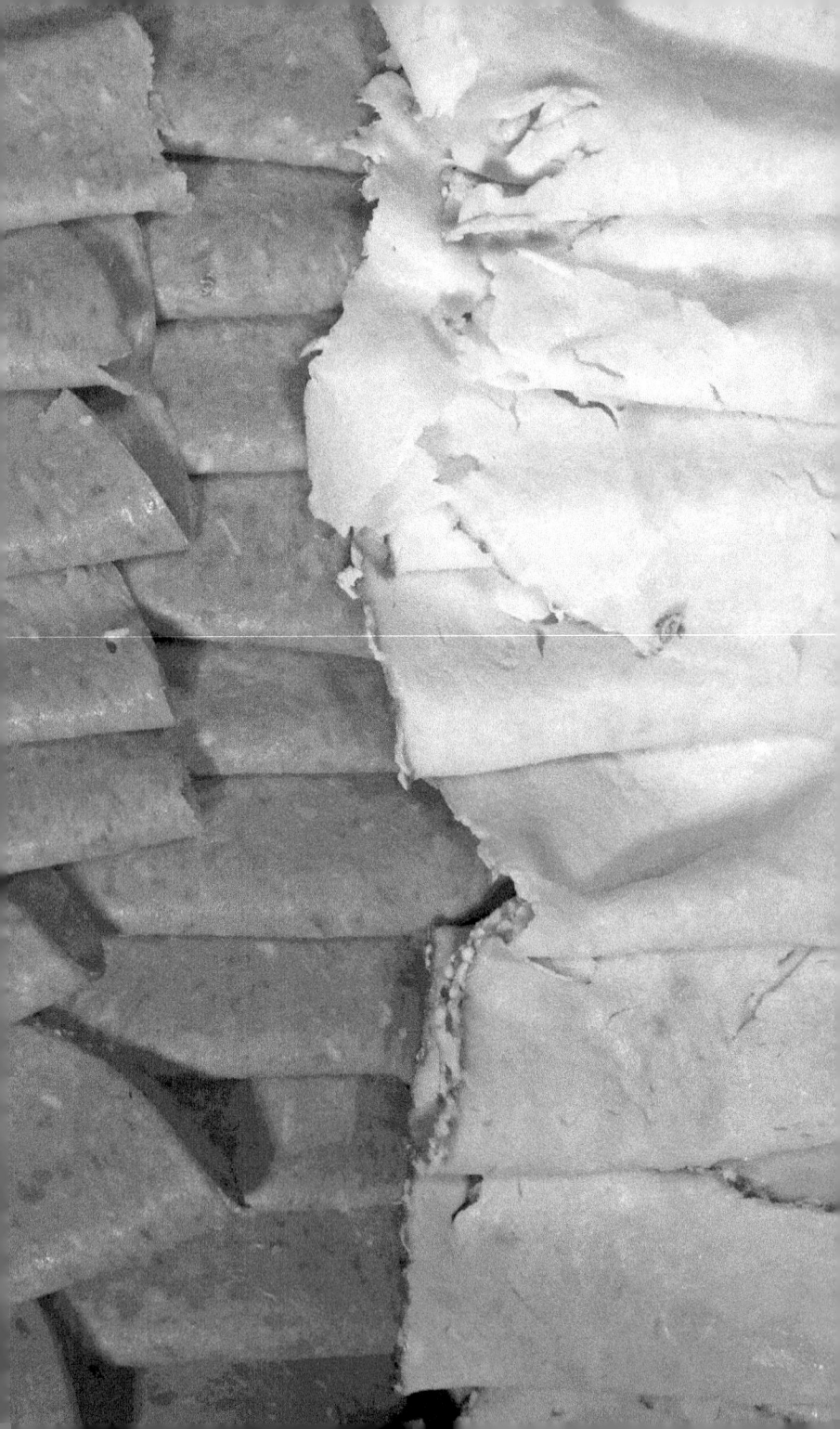

# Deli Meats

 Limit consumption of lunch meats. They contain high amounts of sodium and preservatives which can be harmful to your health.

❖ Sodium nitrate is a preservative used to fight off the harmful bacteria in processed deli meats and to give the meat its fresh looking color. Sodium nitrates can damage blood vessels leading to heart disease and cancer forming cells.

❖ Look for low-sodium and low fat meats.

❖ Avoid meats containing nitrates, MSG (monosodium glutamate), artificial ingredients, and preservatives.

❖ Turkey, chicken, lean ham, and lean roast beef are good low fat options.

# Deli Meats

## *Shopping Tips*

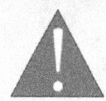 Lunch meats are likely to be exposed to bacteria. Ensure you reseal your packaged meats tightly after each use.

❖ Buy fresh cooked sliced meats when possible.

❖ Avoid bologna, salami, and pastrami – they are high in fat, saturated fat, and sodium.

❖ Be sure to check the expiration date on packaged deli meats.

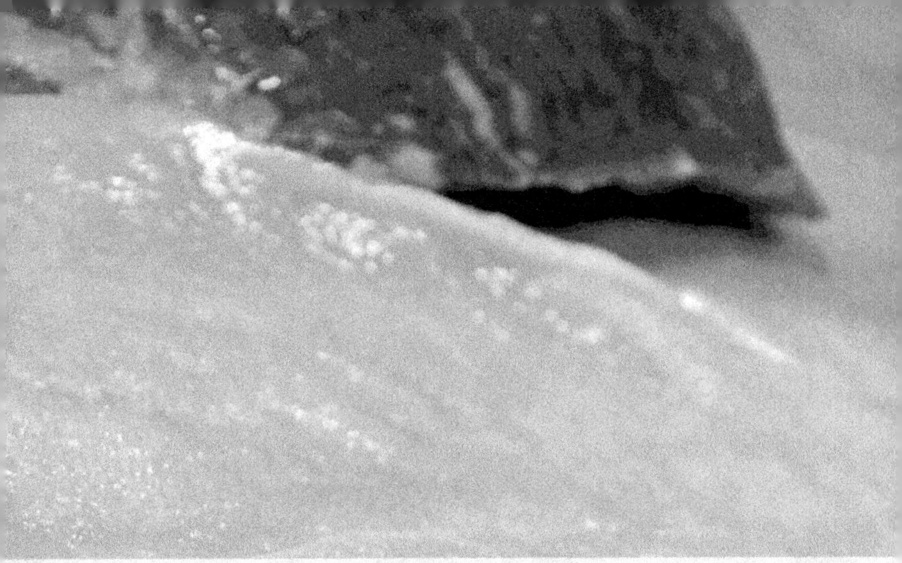

# Meat & Poultry

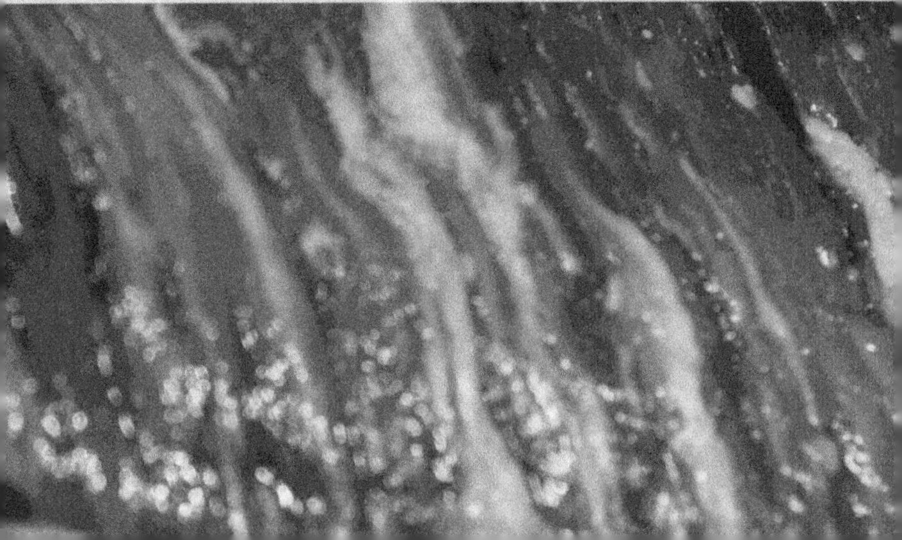

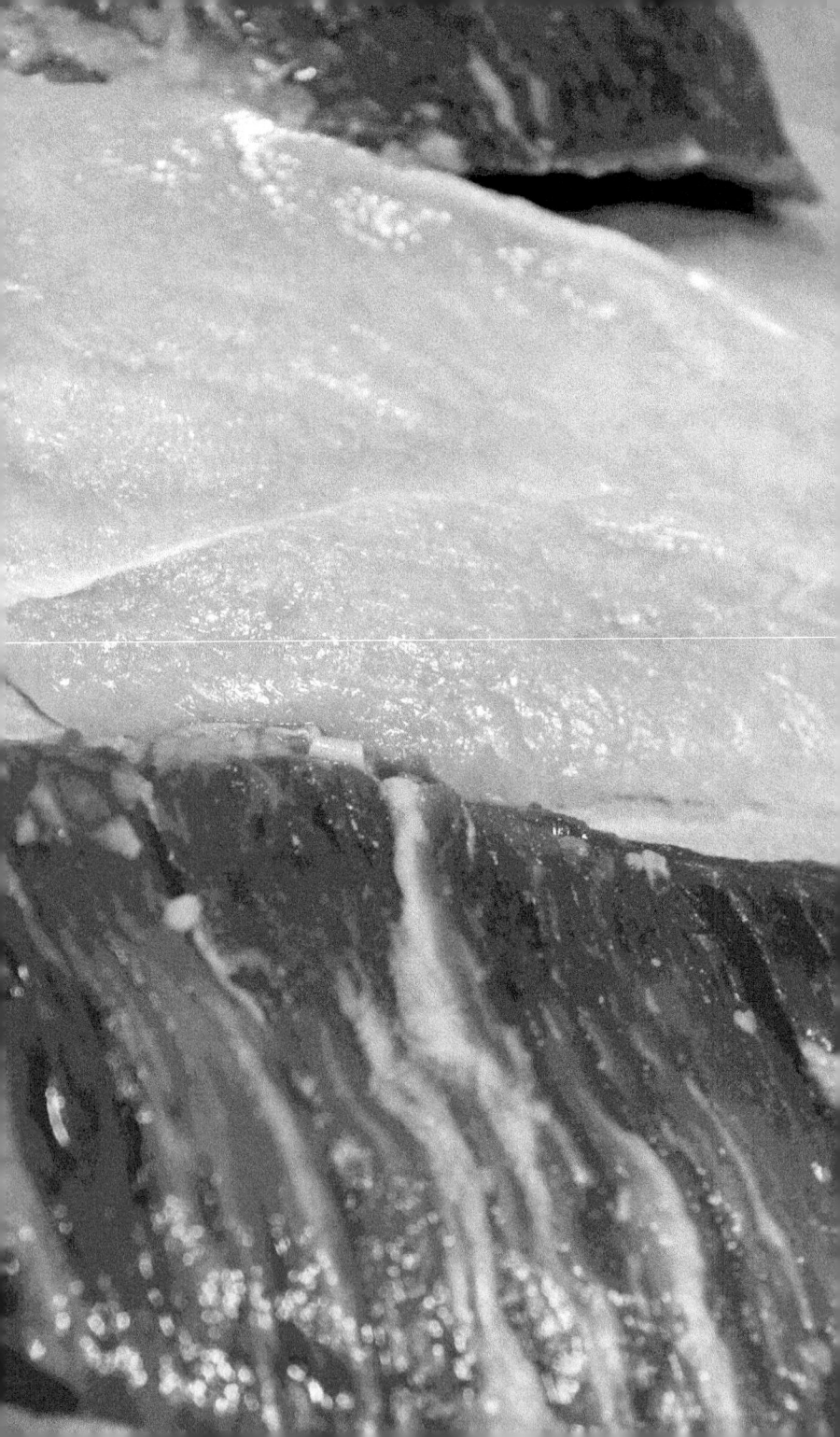

# Meats & Poultry

## *Navigating the Label*

### Cuts of Meat

❖ Lean ground beef: A 3.5 ounce serving contains less than 10 grams of fat, 4.5 grams of saturated fat and 95 mg of cholesterol.

❖ Extra-lean ground beef: A 3.5 ounce serving contains less than 5 grams of fat, 2 grams of saturated fat and 95 mg of cholesterol.

❖ "Choice" or "Select" cuts will have less fat than "prime" cuts.

❖ "Round" and "loin" cuts have the least fat.

❖ Look for ground meat with the lowest fat. Sirloin is typically the leanest cut used in ground meat.

*See the chart on the next page for more information on the leanest cuts of meat.*

**Leanest Cuts of Meat**

### *Poultry*

Skinless chicken or turkey

Chicken or turkey breast

Lean or extra lean ground chicken or turkey

### *Beef*

| | |
|---|---|
| Sirloin tip steak | Eye of round steak |
| Top or bottom round steak | 95% lean ground beef |
| Top sirloin steak | |

### *Veal*

| | |
|---|---|
| Sirloin | Loin chop |
| Rib chop | Top round |

### *Lamb*

| | |
|---|---|
| Arm | Shank of leg |
| Leg | 90% lean ground lamb |
| Loin | |

### *Pork*

| | |
|---|---|
| Pork tenderloin | 90% lean ground pork |
| Boneless sirloin roast | Canadian bacon |
| Boneless top loin chop | |

# Meats & Poultry

## *Navigating the Label*

### Flavoring Meats

❖ Cured meat is meat that has been processed with salt to increase flavor. This is high in sodium and is not an ideal choice.

❖ "Naturally smoked" means meat was roasted or cured in the presence of natural wood.

❖ "Artificially smoked" means flavor on meat was made using chemicals.

❖ "Natural smoked flavor" means flavor was added to enhance taste.

### Raising of Animals

❖ Organic: Animal was not treated with antibiotics or hormones and was fed only organic feed.

❖ Grass fed: Animal grazed in a field rather than being fed out of a trough. Grass fed meats may be higher in omega-3 fatty acids but are not necessarily organic.

# Meats & Poultry

## *Shopping Tips*

 Meat and poultry should be among the last items put in your cart. They should be cold to the touch, not room temperature or warm.

❖ Meat should be bright red when it is fresh.

❖ Packaging should be tightly wrapped without tears or punctures.

❖ There should be no excess liquid or slime in packaging and it should be free of foul odor. Vacuum packed meat should not be bulging.

❖ Check "sell by" date – it should be prepared by or frozen within 2 days of this date.

❖ To freeze, wrap individual pieces in parchment or wax paper. Store in a freezer bag to stay organized.

❖ Store meat on the bottom shelf of the refrigerator to avoid liquids dripping on other food.

❖ Packaged ground meat can contain a variety of cuts of meat. For ground meat that is lowest in fat, pick out your choice of meat and ask the butcher to grind them for you.

❖ When choosing poultry, light meat is lower in cholesterol, fat, and calories than dark meat.

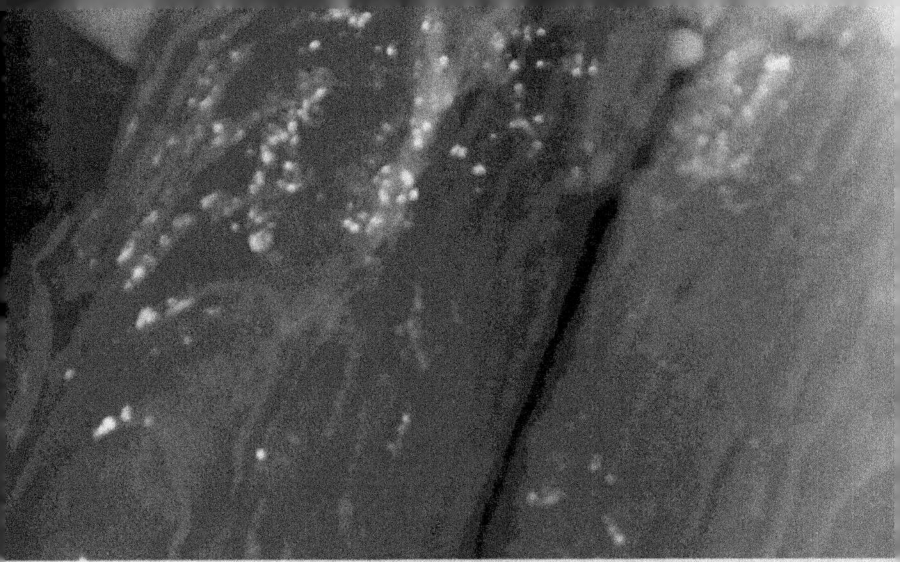

# Fish & Seafood

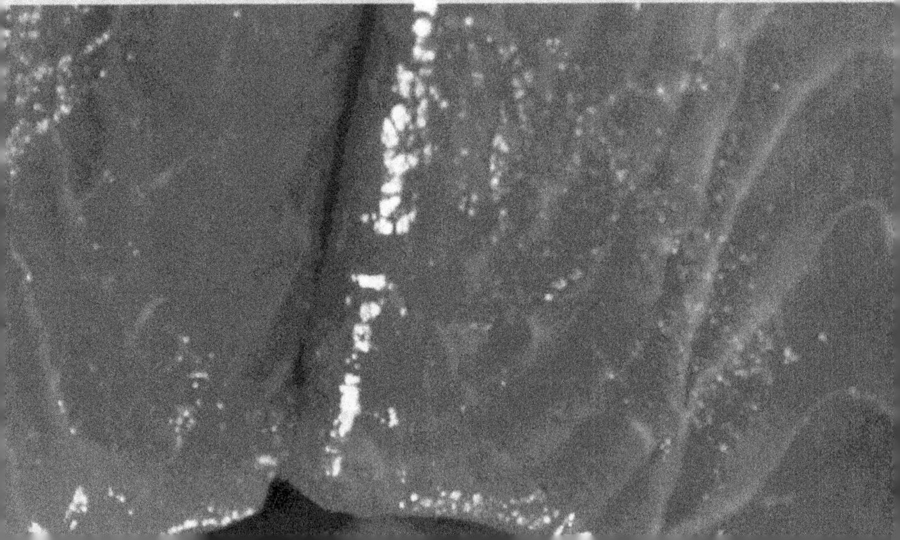

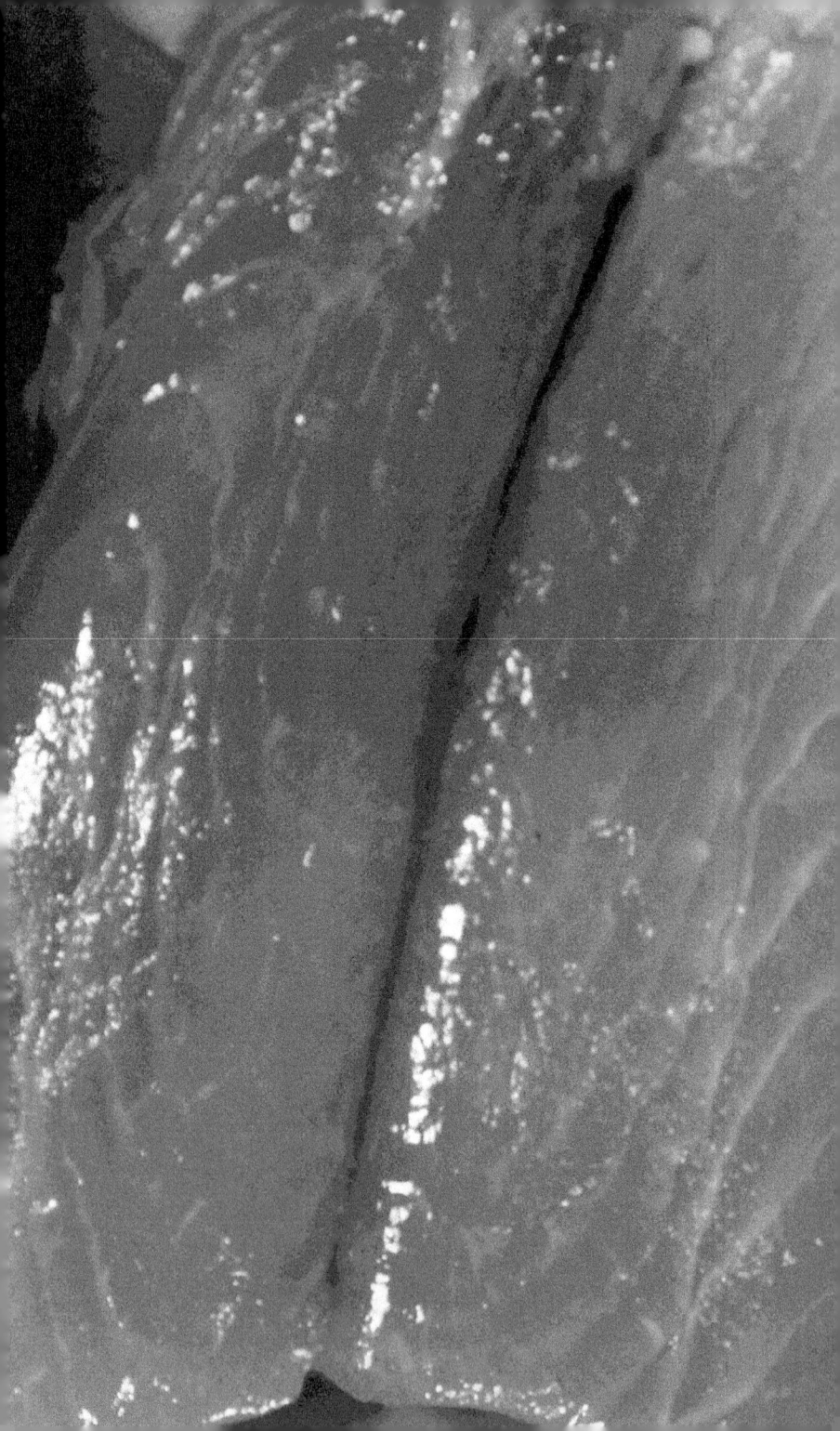

# Fish & Seafood

## *Navigating the Label*

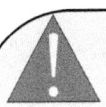 Fish can be high in mercury. Fish not listed on this page may also contain mercury.

It is recommended to consume fish twice a week for health benefits. A typical serving of fish is about 4 ounces for adults. Large amounts of mercury should not be ingested.

Ingesting mercury can be harmful to an unborn baby and a developing child's nervous system. Women who are or may become pregnant, nursing mothers, and young children are urged to avoid fish high in mercury.

### *High in Mercury*

| | |
|---|---|
| Bluefish | Grouper |
| Albacore tuna | Mackerel |
| Chilean sea bass | Yellowfin tuna |

### *Highest in Mercury*

| | |
|---|---|
| Ahi tuna | Orange roughly |
| Bigeye tuna | Shark |
| King mackerel | Swordfish |
| Marlin | Tilefish |

# Fish & Seafood
## *Navigating the Label*

* Canned fish should be packed in water, not oil. This will decrease calories and fat per serving.

* Choose "light" varieties of canned tuna. These have less mercury than "white" varieties.

* Farm-raised fish are usually raised with the use of antibiotics, pesticides, and toxins. They often contain artificial dyes and more fat.

* Wild fish tend to be higher in omega-3 fatty acids and are not treated with pesticides, antibiotics, or artificial dyes. Wild fish may have higher mercury content.

* Salmon, oysters, rainbow trout, striped bass, flounder, sole, Alaskan King Crab, cod halibut, and lobster tail are high in omega-3 fatty acids.

* Shrimp are low in calories and saturated fat, yet high in cholesterol.

# Fish & Seafood

## *Shopping Tips*

❖ Avoid buying cooked fish displayed next to frozen fish; this can cause cross-contamination.

❖ Ask where the fish comes from. The more you know about the fish you purchase, the more you will know about how it was raised, caught, and any possible contaminants.

❖ Save money by purchasing frozen fish rather than fresh fish.

❖ Fresh fish should be stored on ice or in a refrigerator.

❖ Whole fish should have bright eyes, shiny and clean scales, and bright red gills.

❖ Fresh fillets should be bright and/or shiny metallic.

❖ There should be no overpowering aroma or milky liquid, only clear liquid if any.

❖ Check freshness by pressing fish. The indentation from your finger should disappear when fresh.

❖ The shell of clams or mussels should be shut. An open shell means it is beginning to spoil.

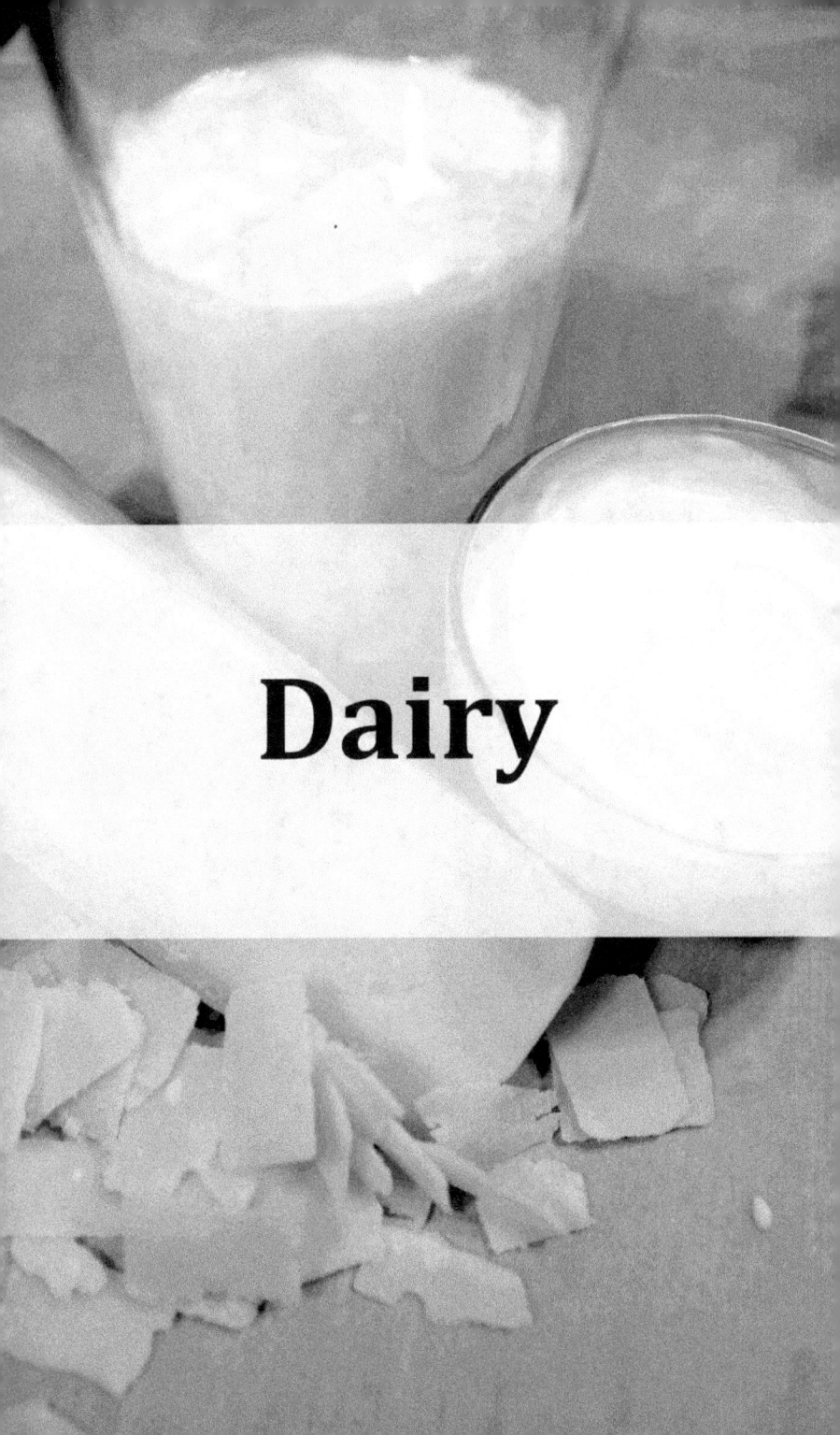

# Dairy

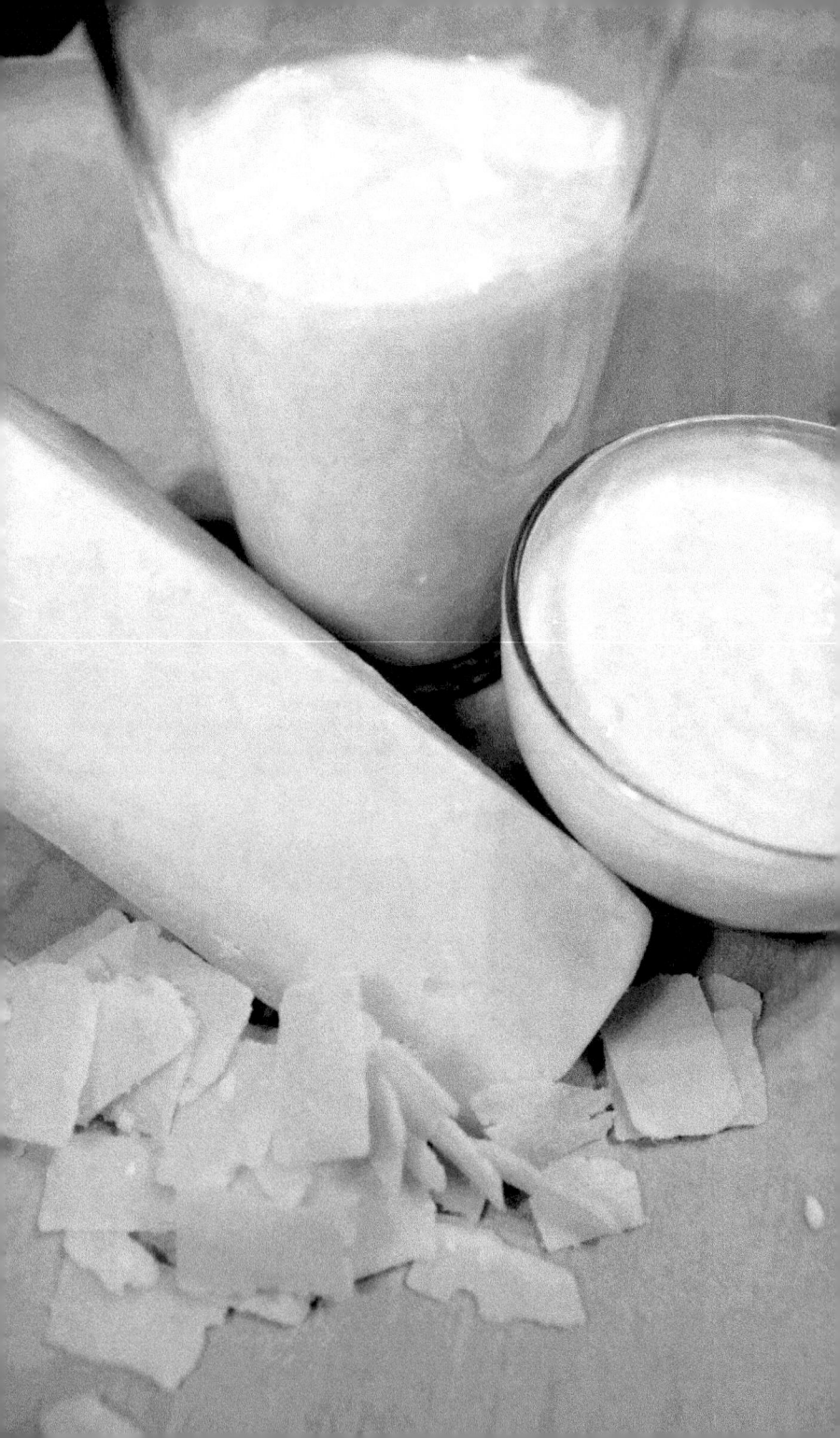

# Dairy
## *Navigating the Label*

**Milk**

❖ Percent fat does not refer to the percentage of calories in milk from fat. It refers to how much weight from fat contributes to the overall weight of the milk.

❖ Whole milk refers to milk in its fullest state in which no fat is removed.

❖ Fat free, 1%, and 2% milk go through processing to remove the cream in order to reduce fat and calories. They have the same amount of protein, calcium, and vitamins A & D as whole milk.

❖ Organic milk comes from dairy farms that use organic fertilizers and pesticides and from cows that were not treated with hormones.

**Milk Processing**

❖ There are 3 processing steps that milk typically goes through before being sold in stores: pasteurization, homogenization, and fortification.

❖ Pasteurization is a process which extends the shelf-life of milk. Milk is heated to destroy microorganisms without harming the nutrient content.

❖ Homogenization is a process which combines the milk fat evenly throughout the milk to prevent separation and to create an even texture.

# Dairy

**Milk Processing** *continued*

❖ <u>Fortification</u> is used to increase nutrients or to replace nutrients lost in processing. Most milk products are fortified with vitamin D and vitamin A.

**Milk Alternatives**

❖ Lactose-free milk is cow's milk that has been treated with lactase, an enzyme which helps break down the lactose in milk.

❖ Soy milk is a great source of protein but contains less vitamin D and calcium than cow's milk. Look for soymilk that is fortified with these nutrients.

❖ Rice milk is made with rice, rice syrup, and sweetener. It contains twice as much carbohydrates as cow's milk and is low in vitamin D and calcium. Be aware of carbohydrate content and choose fortified options.

❖ Almond milk is typically lower in calories and protein than cow's milk.

**Yogurt**

❖ Look for yogurt high in protein (14-17 grams), low in fat (no more than 3 grams) and low in sugar.

❖ Greek yogurt has more protein, less sugar, and less carbohydrates than other yogurts.

# Dairy

## *Navigating the Label*

### Yogurt *continued*

❖ All yogurts, even plain, will have 12 grams of sugar from lactose. This is the naturally occurring carbohydrate in dairy products.

❖ Look for brands using live active cultures. These are microorganisms that are beneficial for your digestion and regulating your system.

### Cheese

❖ Cheese can be a good source of calcium. Look for varieties that are at least 15% of the daily value.

❖ Choose hard cheese that has 3 grams or less fat per serving.

❖ Check serving sizes before enjoying. Serving sizes are often small so calories and fat can add up quickly.

# Dairy

❖ Remember to check the expiration date on all dairy products. You want to use before the date printed on the container for the freshest product.

❖ Soy and almond milk may be sweetened or flavored and can be high in sugar. Look for unsweetened versions.

❖ Choose low fat or fat free plain yogurt. Adding your own fruit will save you a lot of added sugar.

❖ Look for reduced fat or light cheese options for lower fat and calorie content.

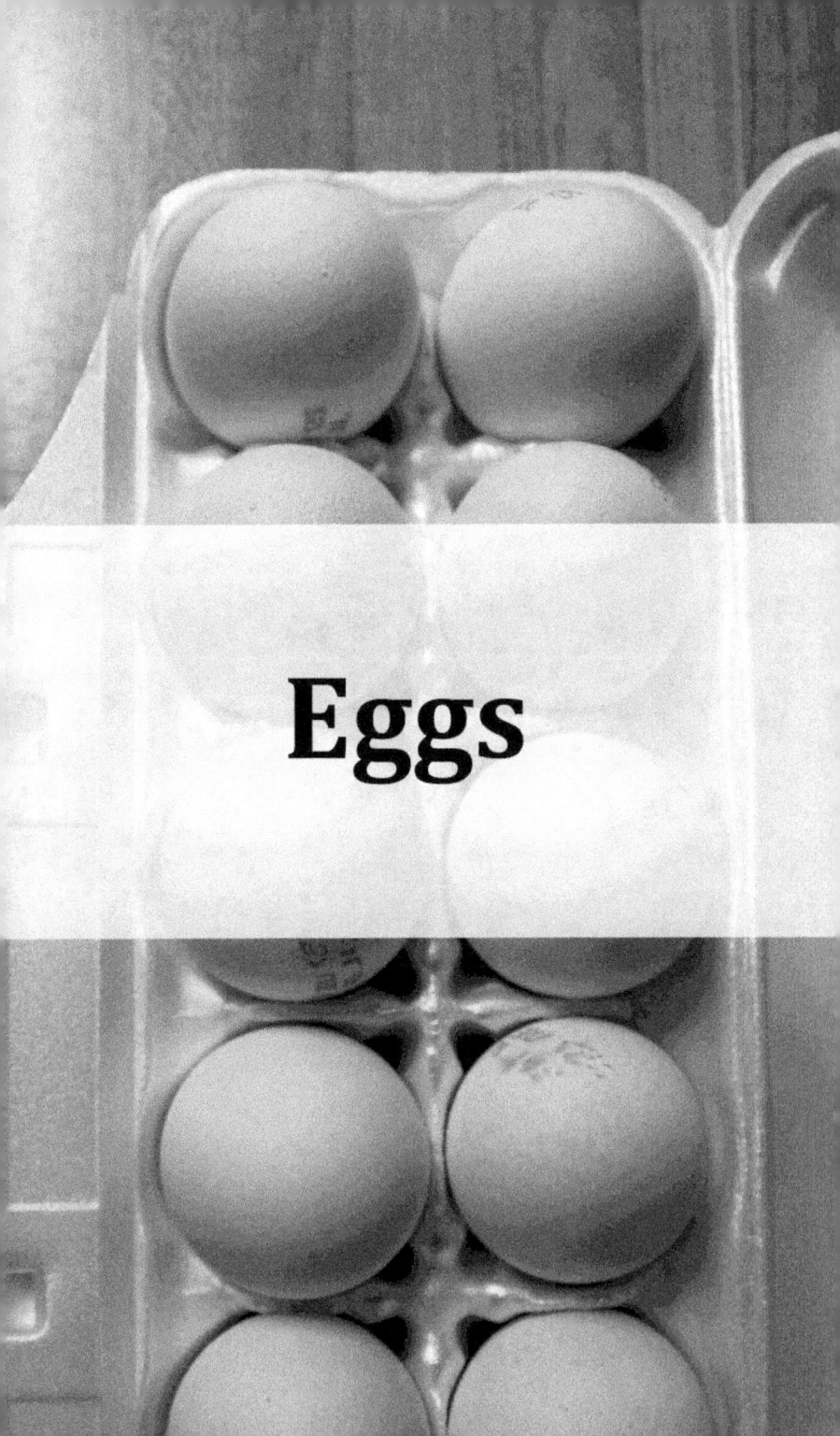

Eggs

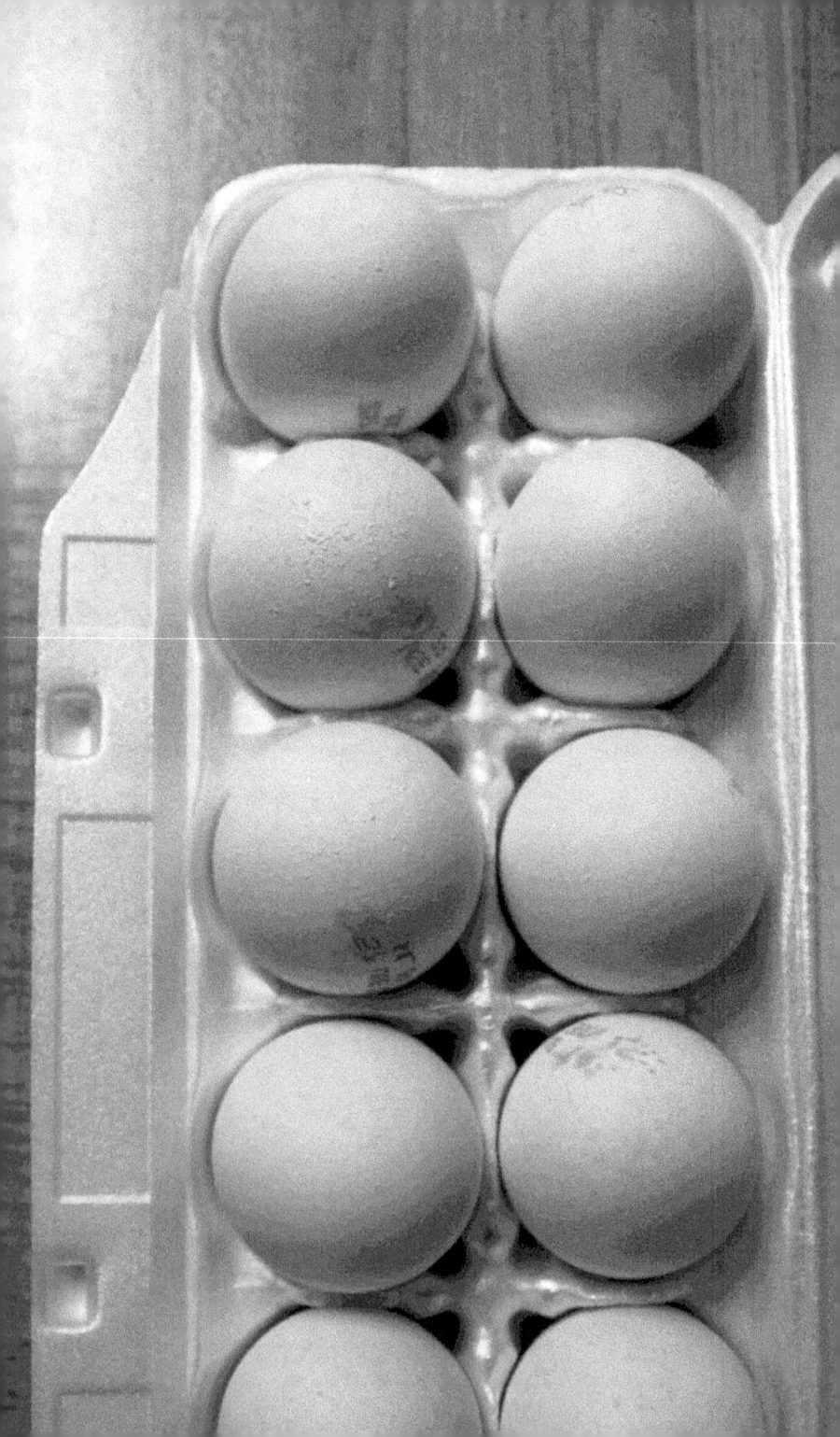

# Eggs

## *Navigating the Label*

### Types of Eggs

❖ U.S. Grade AA and U.S. Grade A: Eggs have whites and yolks that stand high and are practically free from defects. Shells should be clean and unbroken.

❖ US. Grade B: Eggs have thinner whites and wider yolks. The shells are unbroken but may have slight stains.

❖ White and brown eggs have the same nutrition content. The difference is related to what color physical features the hen had. Hens with dark features lay brown eggs while hens with lighter features lay white eggs.

### Labeling Terms

❖ Organic: Hens are raised on feed that is free of pesticides, fertilizers, and antibiotics. These hens are typically cage-free and given outdoor access.

❖ Omega-3: Hens are raised on feed that contains higher omega-3 fatty acids.

❖ Pasteurized: Eggs are heated just enough to kill pathogens. These eggs may be used in recipes which call for raw egg.

# Eggs

❖ Eggs come in sizes: small, medium, large, extra-large, and jumbo. Recipes typically call for large eggs.

❖ If you plan on substituting egg whites for whole eggs, keep in mind that 2 egg whites is equal to 1 whole egg.

❖ Liquid egg whites are a lower fat, lower cholesterol alternative to whole eggs. You can find them in cartons near the whole eggs.

❖ Be sure to check the carton of eggs before purchasing to ensure the eggs are not cracked.

❖ Terms such as "natural", "antibiotic-free" or "hormone-free" don't mean much when on egg cartons.

❖ "Natural" is an unregulated term for eggs and hens used to produce eggs aren't normally treated with hormones or antibiotics. Avoid spending more on these empty claims.

# Grains

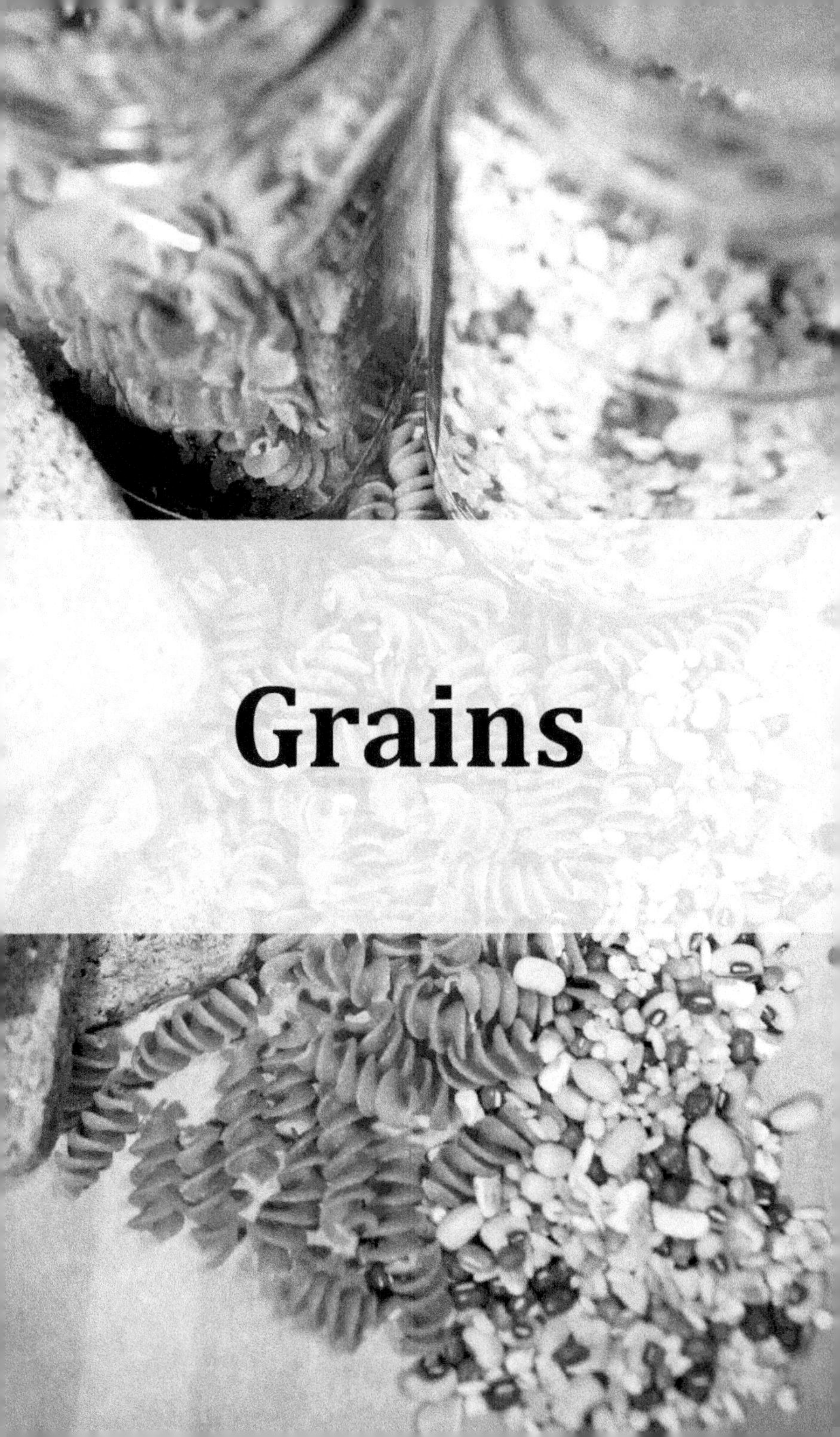

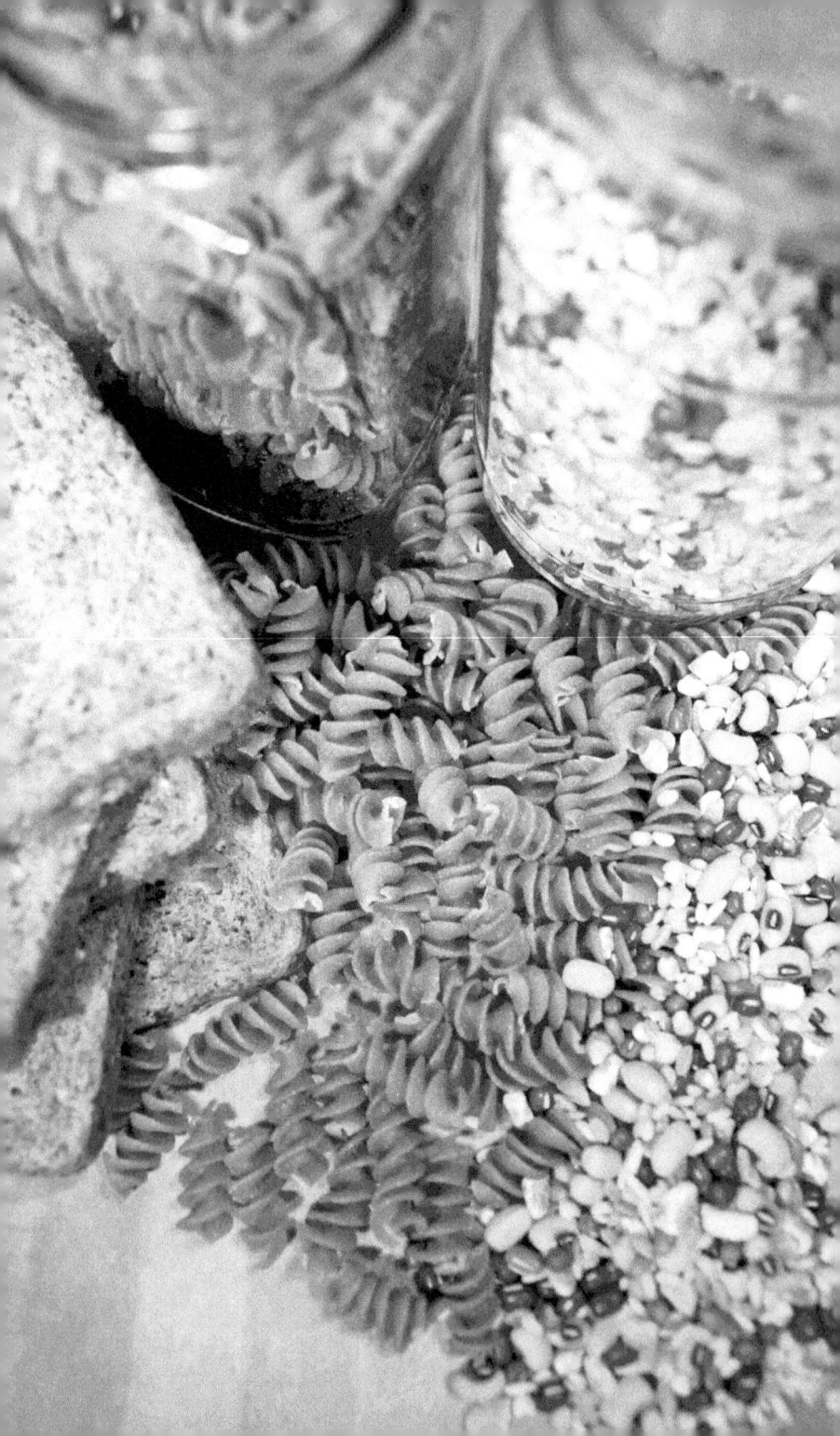

# Grains

## *Navigating the Label*

❖ When shopping for whole grain products, look for the word "whole" before the grain on the ingredient list. If it says "enriched" or "refined" it is not a whole grain product.

❖ It is recommended that adults eat at least 48 grams of whole grains each day.

❖ Whole grain products will contain more fiber than refined or enriched products. Check the nutrition label for fiber content of at least 2 grams.

❖ Do not get fooled by misleading labels. These appealing terms are not equivalents to whole grain: multigrain, stone ground, 100% wheat.

❖ Some products will have the Whole Grain Stamp to help you know if it is a whole grain product.

> › The 100% Whole Grain Stamp indicates that all of its grain ingredients are whole grains.

> › The Basic Stamp indicates that the product contains at least 8 grams of whole grains, but may contain refined grains as well.

# Grains

❖ Whole grain products should contain at least 2 grams of dietary fiber per serving.

  › "Good Source of Fiber" or "High in Fiber" means there is 2.5 to 5 grams of fiber per serving.

  › "Excellent Source of Fiber" indicates there is greater than 5 grams of fiber per serving.

❖ Packaged bread tend to have hidden sodium. Look for loaves with lower sodium content. Try finding options with 140 milligrams or less per serving.

❖ Be aware of bread with added sweetness such as "honey wheat" as they may contain more sugar than other breads.

# Grains

## *Shopping Tips*

### *Examples of Whole Grains*

| | |
|---|---|
| Whole grain barley | Rolled oats |
| Brown rice | Whole oats |
| Buckwheat | Quinoa |
| Bulgur | Wheatberries |
| Whole grain corn | Whole rye or rye berries |
| Farro | Whole grain sorghum |
| Millet | Whole wheat |
| Oatmeal | Wild rice |

❖ Aim for buying mostly whole grain breads, pastas, and grains. Refined grains generally should be kept to a minimum.

❖ You will find many brands of pastas, breads, and grains. Simply choose options that have "whole" grains listed as the primary ingredient and those that contain 2 or more grams of dietary fiber per serving.

❖ Don't be surprised to find rice pasta, quinoa pasta, and more in supermarkets. These varieties are typically gluten-free and have a different taste and texture than wheat pasta.

❖ Be aware of other common confusions about whole grains. For example, dark breads are not necessarily whole grain.

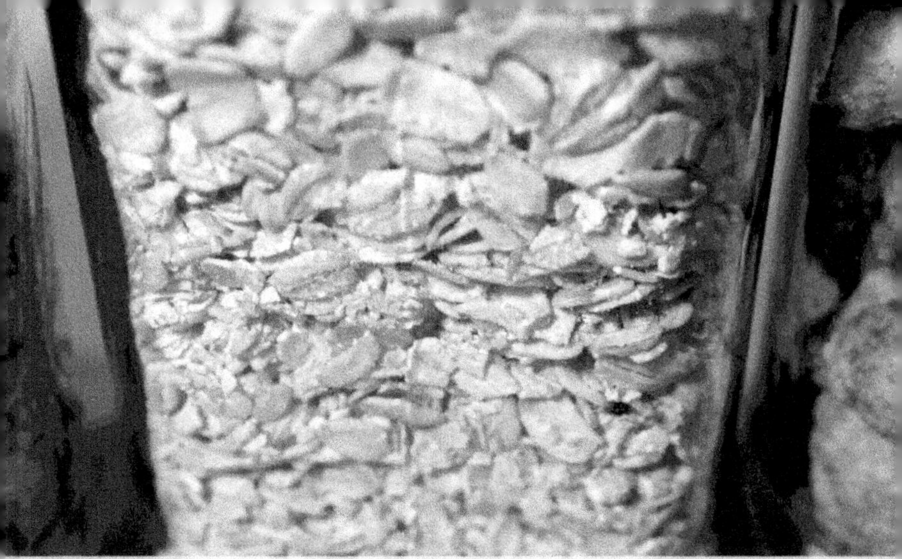

# Hot & Cold Cereal

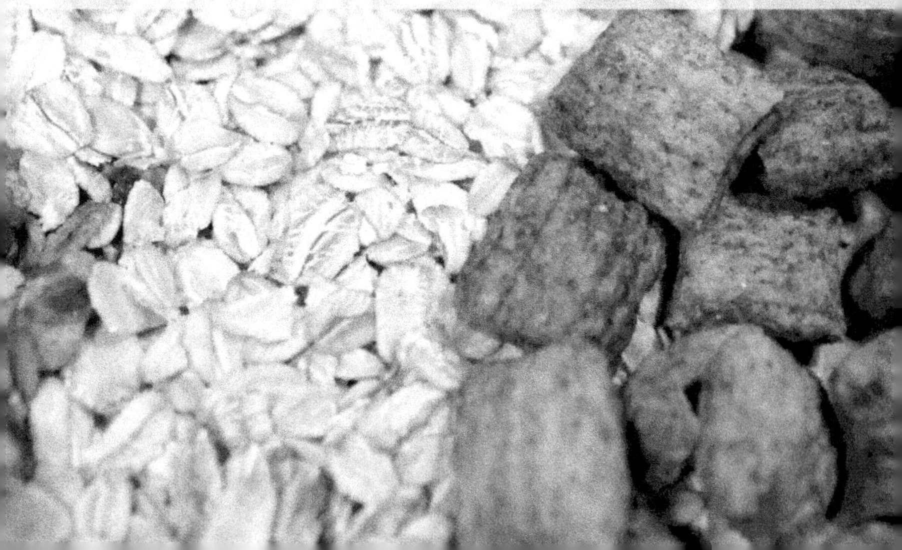

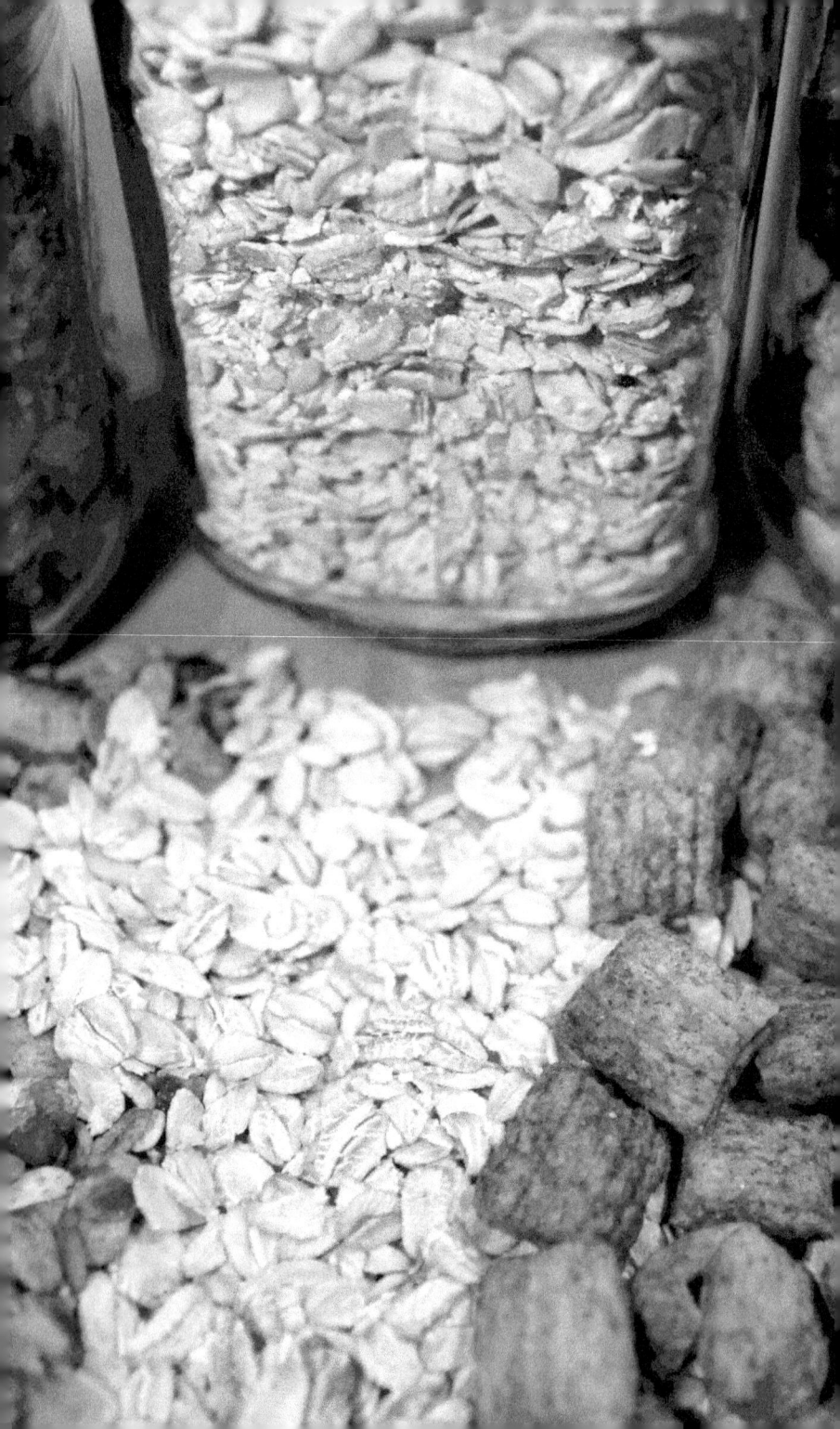

# Hot & Cold Cereal

## *Navigating the Label*

 Cereal can be a nutritious breakfast to start your day but be mindful of your serving sizes. It can be easy to go over the serving size listed on the package without noticing, and you will be eating more calories, fat, and sugar than intended.

❖ Choose cereals that have the first ingredient listed as a "whole" grain.

❖ Choose cereals with at least 3 grams of fiber and 3 grams or less fat per serving.

❖ Choose options with 6 or less grams of sugar per serving. Sugar may be listed in the ingredients as sucrose, honey, corn syrup, fructose, molasses, fruit juice sweeteners, or malt syrup.

❖ Granola and granola cereals may seem like a sound breakfast choice but be aware of the nutrition label. These products often contain more added sugar and fat than breakfast cereals.

❖ For a cereal with adequate nutrition to start your day, look for hot and cold cereals that are made with whole grains, high in fiber, and low in sugar, fat, calories, and sodium.

# Hot & Cold Cereal

## Shopping Tips

❖ Opt for "plain", "original", or "unsweetened" versions of oatmeal. Flavored and sweetened varieties contain added sugar and fat.

❖ Cereal with added fruit will have a high sugar content. Keep in mind that with premixed cereals, you should look out for artificial colors and flavors.

❖ Buy the plain versions of cereal and add your own fresh fruit and other flavors. Try mixing apples and ground cinnamon into plain cereal for a healthy version of a popular prepacked flavor.

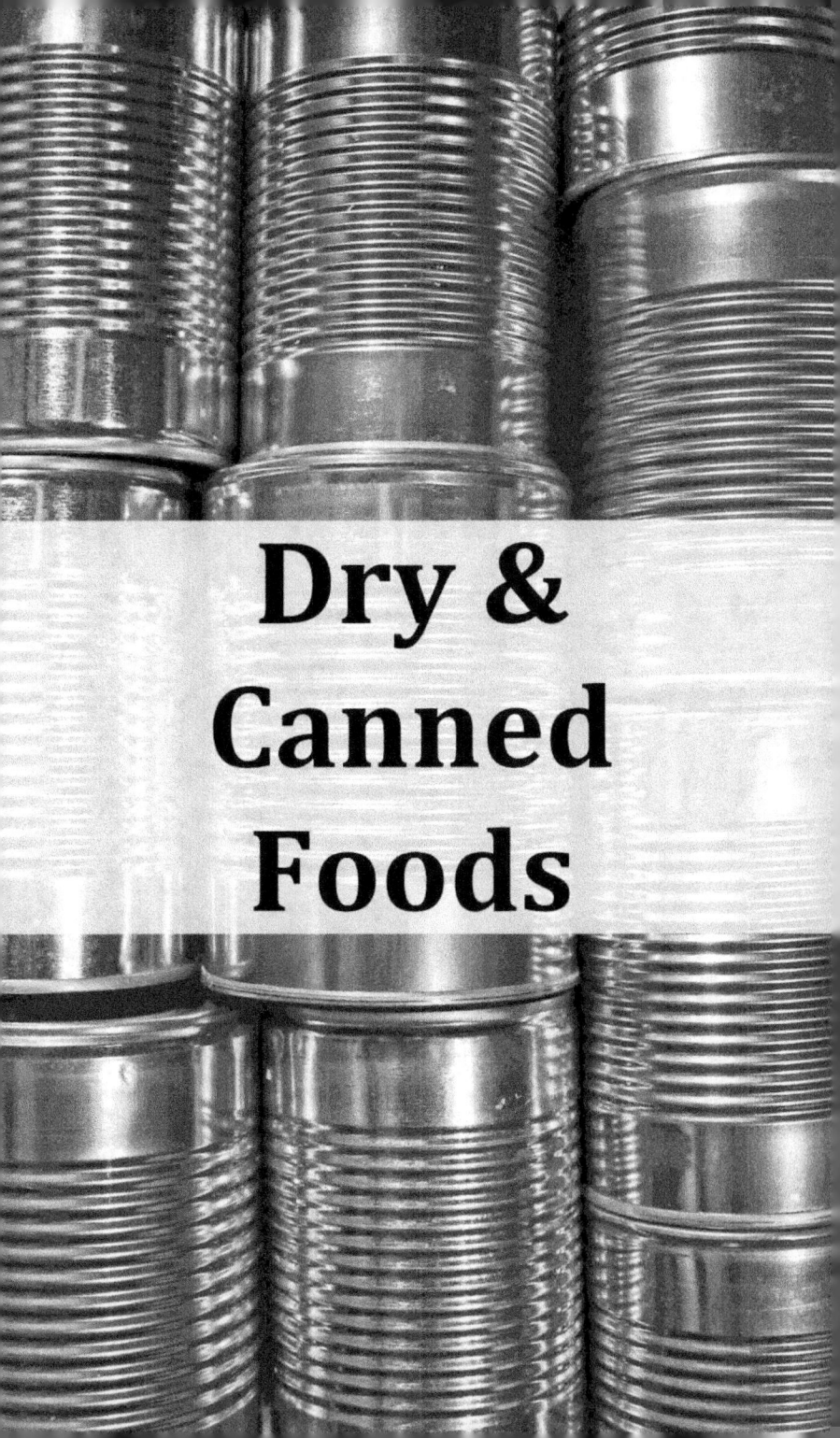

# Dry & Canned Foods

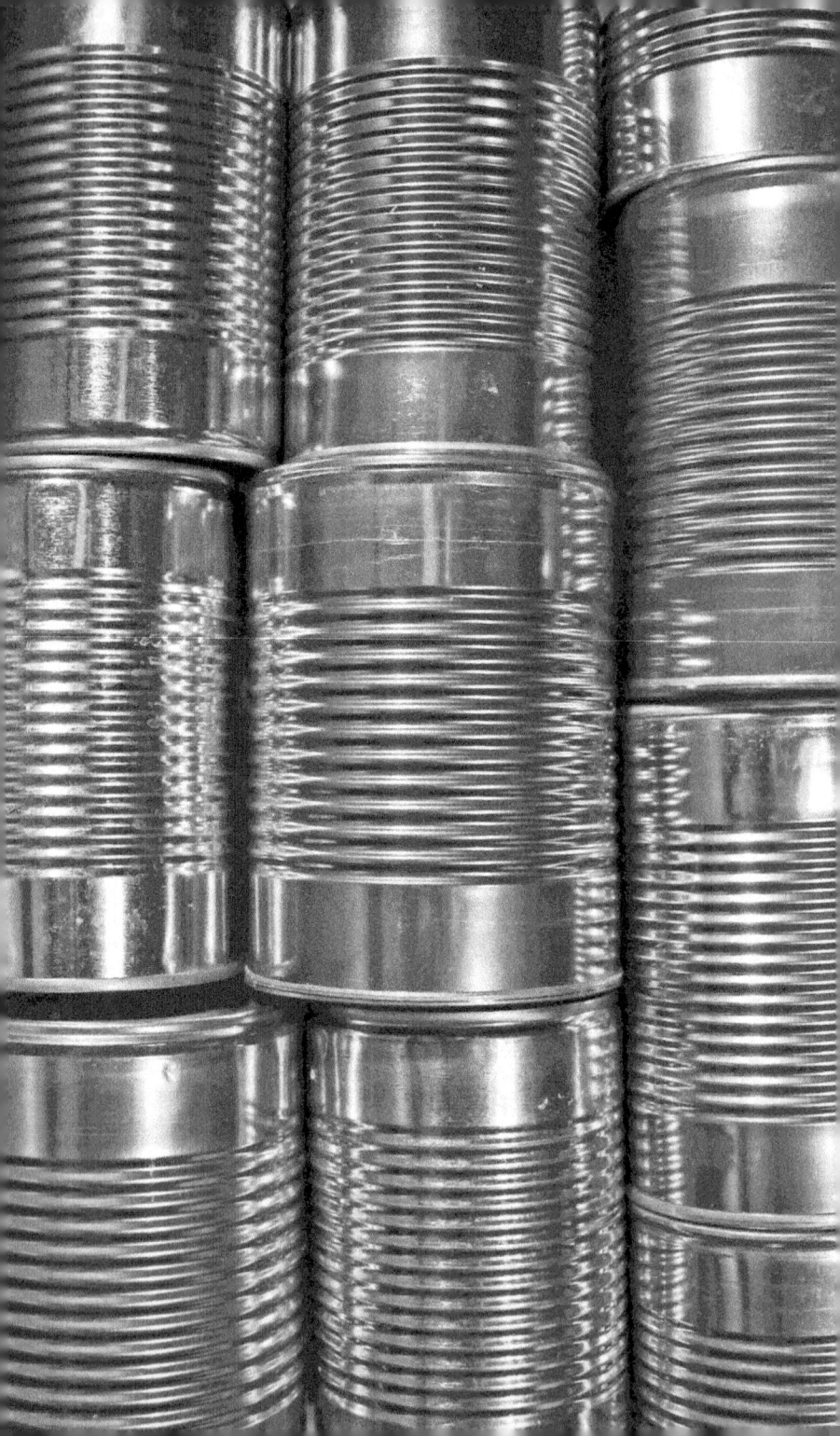

# Dry & Canned Foods

## *Navigating the Label*

### All Canned Foods

❖ Choose canned foods with no added salt and less than 140 milligrams of sodium per serving.

❖ Read the fine print if you have food allergies or restrictions. Many vegetables soups are made with chicken or beef stock. Some soups may contain whey, a dairy component, or wheat flour which contains gluten.

❖ Choose products packed in water instead of oil or juice.

❖ Avoid canned foods which contain corn syrup.

### Fruits & Vegetables

❖ Canned fruit should be prepared in water instead of syrup or natural juice, which increase the sugar content.

❖ Canned vegetables should be labeled "low sodium" or "no salt added" for reduced sodium options. Always rinse canned vegetables before eating.

### Soups

❖ Soups containing beans will be higher in fiber and contain plant-based protein.

❖ Opt for "reduced sodium" soups.

# Dry & Canned Foods

## *Navigating the Label*

**Beans, Legumes, Nuts, & Seeds**

❖ Beans and legumes are available both in dry and canned. Dry beans require more time to prepare.

❖ If using canned beans, choose options without added salt, fat, or sugar. Always rinse your beans well before using.

❖ Look for raw, unsalted nuts and seeds. Varieties with added flavors also have added sodium and sugar.

# Dry & Canned Foods

## *Shopping Tips*

 Do not buy cans that have dents, bulges, or leaks. Damaged cans such as these indicate possible growth of bacteria which can result in foodborne illness.
Always check the "sell by" date for freshness.

❖ Soups can be made to be more filling and to feed more people by adding in vegetables and beans.

❖ For increased fiber, choose bean or split pea soups.

❖ Avoid refried beans which contain lard or partially hydrogenated fats. Fat-free varieties are usually available instead.

❖ Choose ground or milled flax seed for maximum nutrient benefits.

❖ Mind your serving sizes to keep calories and fat in control.

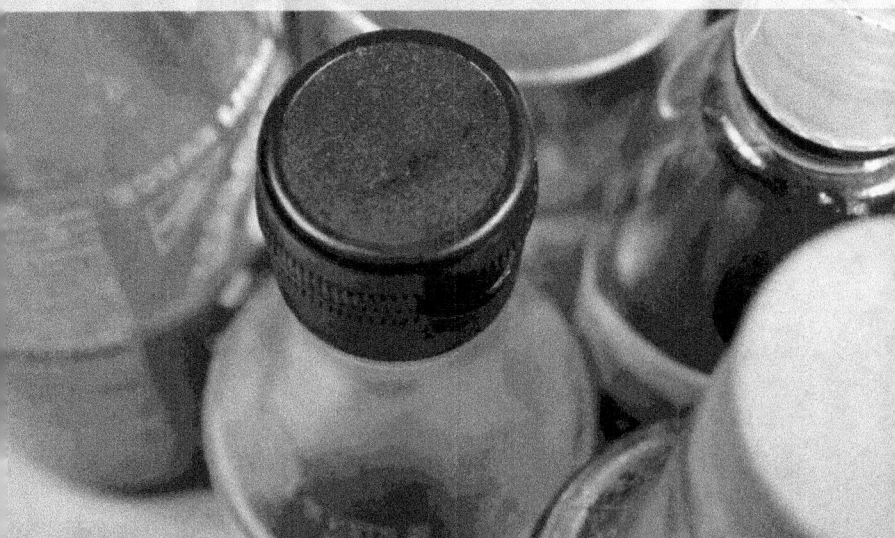

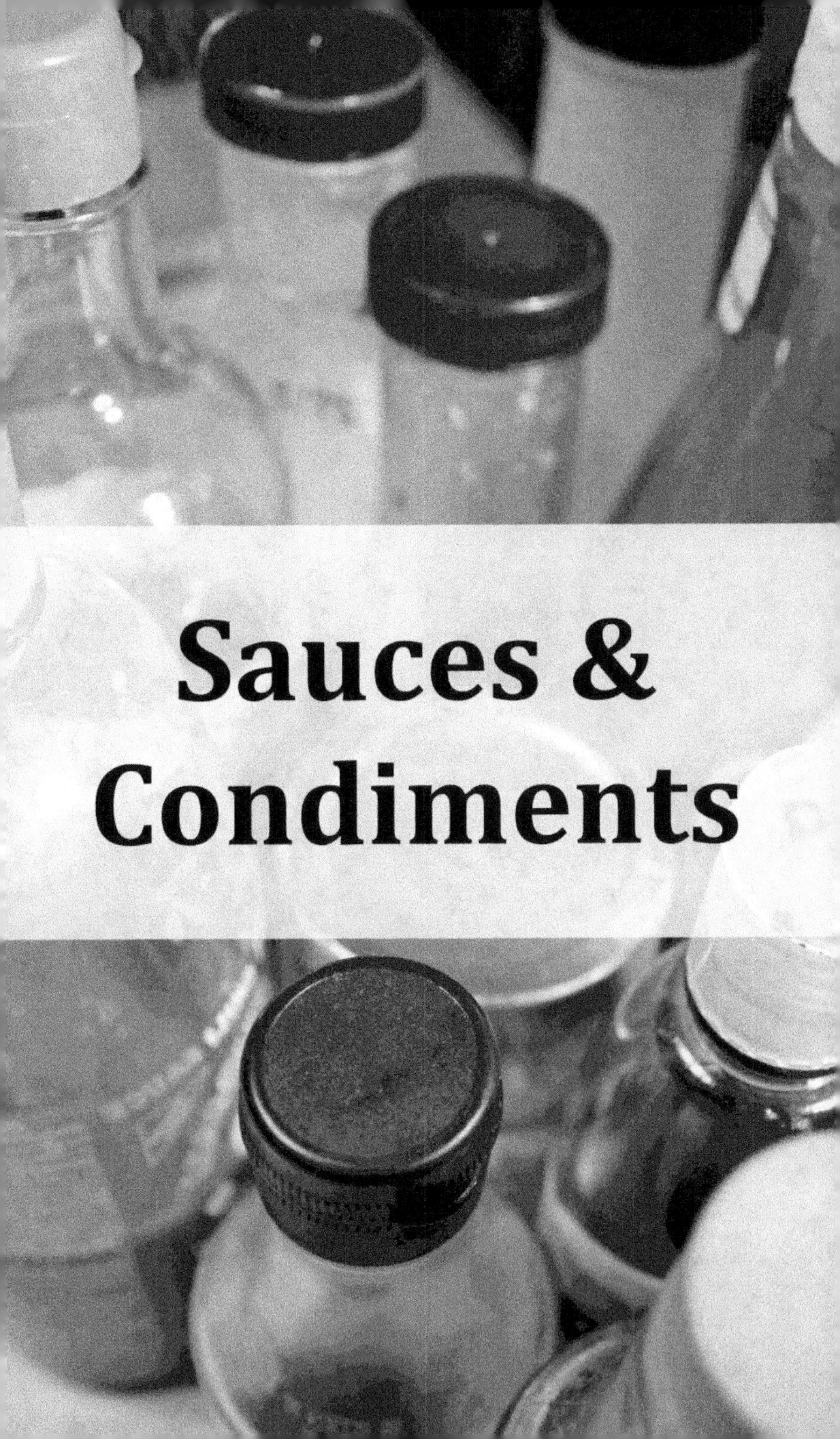

# Sauces & Condiments

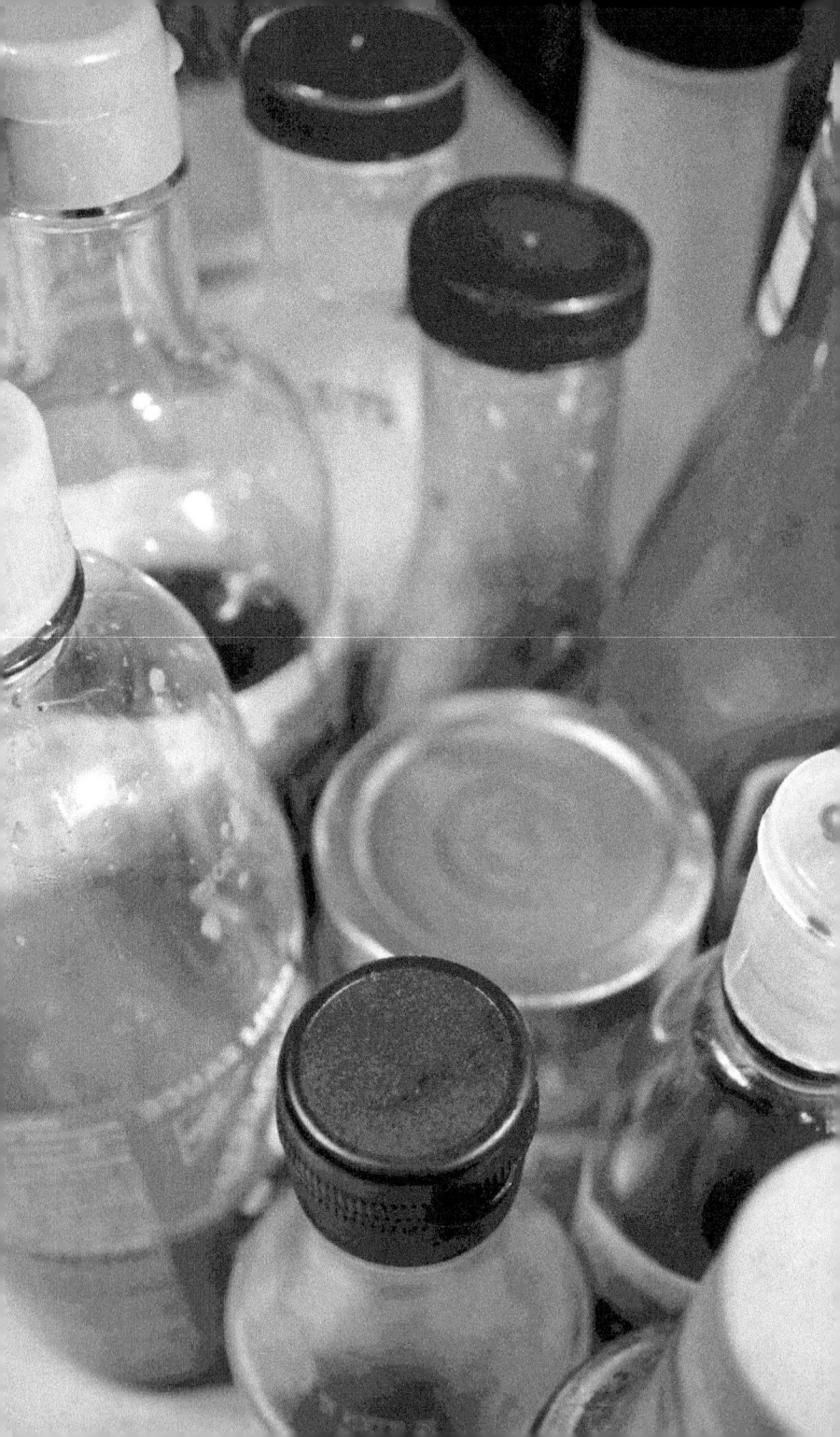

# Sauces & Condiments
## *Navigating the Label*

### Sauces

❖ Sauces such as marinades, dipping sauces, and tomato-based pasta sauces should contain less than 140 milligrams of sodium per serving.

❖ Choose tomato-based pasta sauces or marinara sauce over cream based sauces such as Alfredo sauce. Cream based sauces are high in fat and calories.

### Salad Dressing

❖ Opt for oil-based dressings over cream-based dressings which contain more fat and calories.

❖ Avoid dressings containing sulfites, MSG (monosodium glutamate), and artificial flavor and colors.

### Jam & Jelly

❖ Look for "natural" spreads that are made with real fruit.

❖ Fruit should be first or second on the list and juice concentrates should be the only sweetener on the list, not high fructose corn syrup.

❖ A tablespoon of jam should contain no more than 40 calories.

# Sauces & Condiments
## *Navigating the Label*

### Nut Butter

❖ Look for "natural" spreads that are made with real nuts and without added sugars.

❖ Avoid nut butters which contain hydrogenated oils and trans fat.

### Oil

❖ Choose unsaturated oils over saturated oils. Unsaturated fats are "good" fats.

❖ Monounsaturated oils include olive oil and canola oil which are best for heart health.

❖ Polyunsaturated oils include safflower oil, corn oil, and cottonseed oil.

### Butter & Margarine

❖ Butter is naturally high in saturated fat and cholesterol.

❖ Whipped butter is whipped with air to make it light and fluffy. It contains less fat than regular butter.

❖ Light buttery spread contains no cholesterol and is 50% lower in fat than regular butter.

❖ Margarine contains no cholesterol but is hydrogenated. If you choose margarine, look for versions made without hydrogenated fats.

# Sauces & Condiments

## *Shopping Tips*

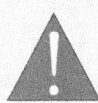 Be aware that just because there is less fat in a product that it may not be better for you.

Fat-free does not mean sugar-free or calorie-free.

❖ Measure out condiments before adding them to your food. This will help you be mindful of serving sizes.

❖ Compare labels and choose salad dressings that are flavored with a variety of herbs and flavors and with the least amount of fat.

❖ Healthier condiments include yellow or spicy mustard, hot sauce, vinegar, extra virgin olive oil, and natural herbs or spices, and low-salt seasoning blends.

❖ Hummus can be a great substitute for other condiments and spreads. Avoid versions with any artificial flavorings.

❖ Choose natural nut butters without added salt and sugar.

❖ Avoid products with trans fats. This includes products which have hydrogenated or partially hydrogenated fats.

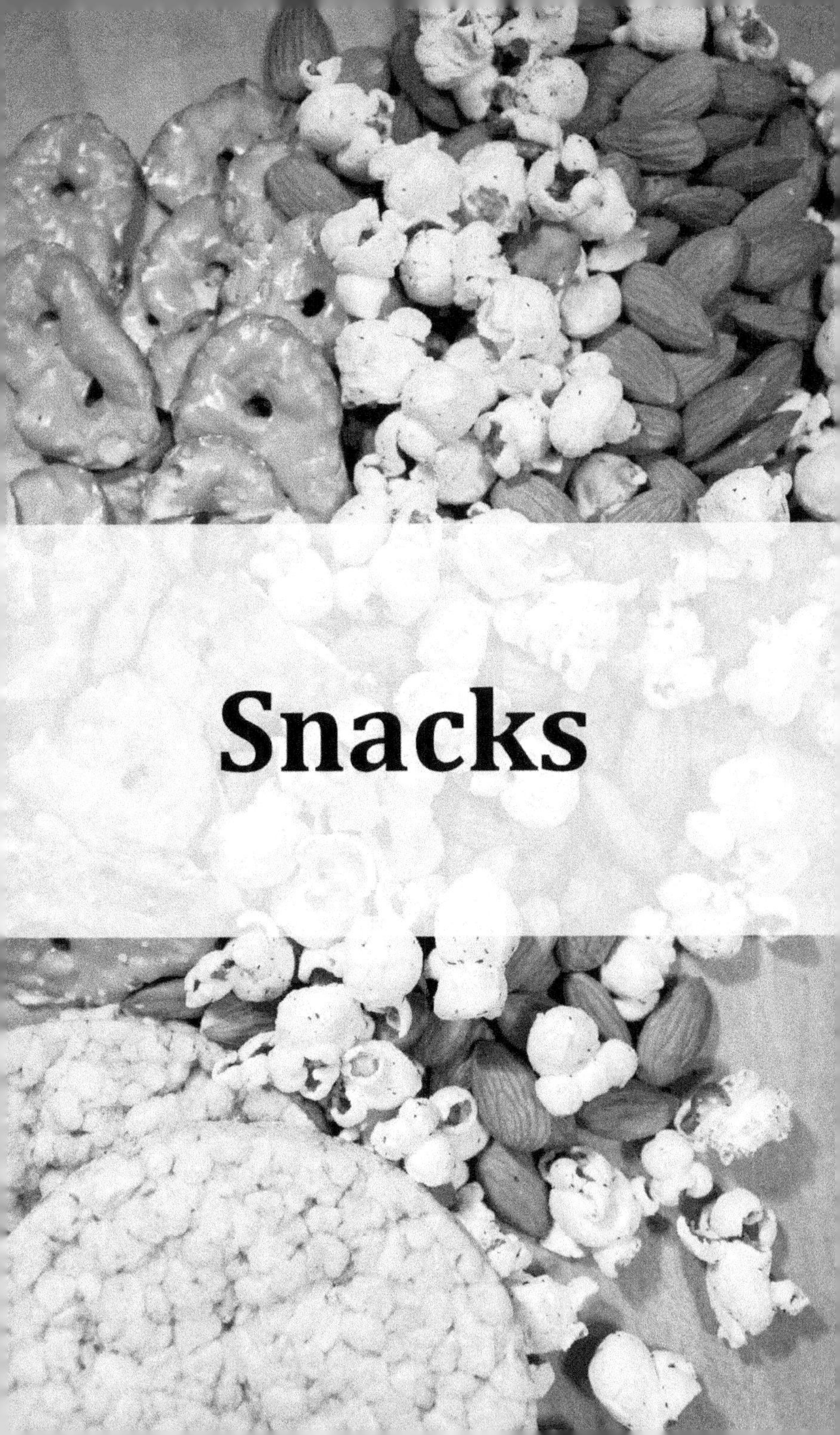

# Snacks

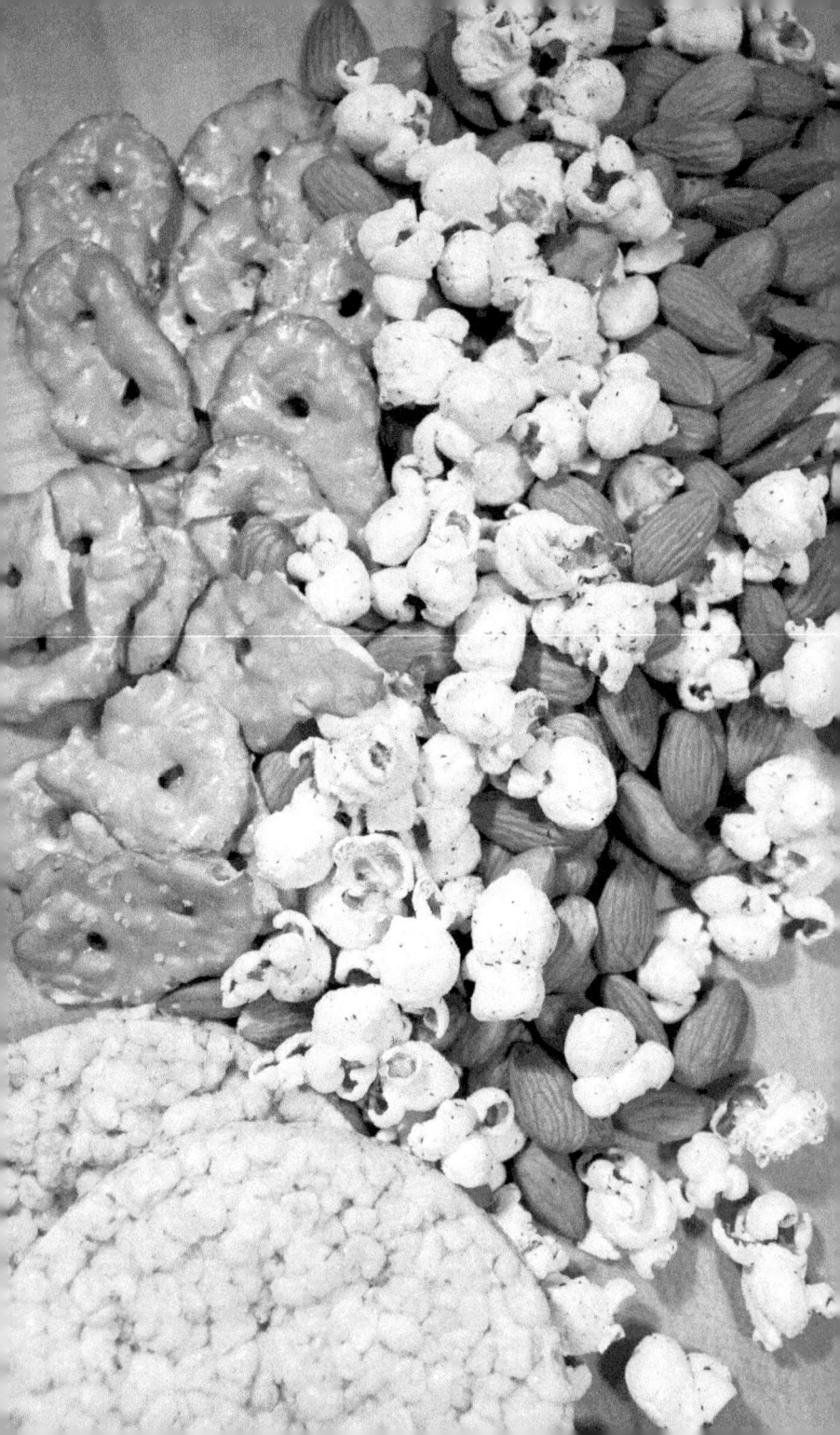

# Snacks

## *Navigating the Label*

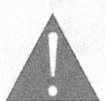 Check the serving size of snacks before eating. Usually a serving size is less than you would expect and calories and fat can quickly add up. Portion out just one serving size of the snack and put the rest away.

❖ Be aware of "trans fat" which will be listed on the nutrition label. Trans fats raise the "bad" cholesterol which can increase your risk of heart disease. Look out for "partially hydrogenated oils" which are also an indicator of trans fats.

❖ Check the sodium content and the ingredients list for hidden sodium sources. Most packages and snack foods are high in salt.

❖ Choose snacks with a maximum of 150-200 calories per serving.

❖ Opt for raw and unsalted nuts.

❖ For snacks that are mainly grains, such as crackers, check the ingredient list for "whole" grains.

❖ "Veggie" snacks don't always mean they are healthier. They are often fried just like regular potato chips.

❖ "Baked" chips are usually lower in fat than fried chips. It is still important to look out for added sodium.

# Snacks

❖ Chips made from whole grains, sweet potato, and soy are often more nutritious than chips made from white potatoes. It is still important to be mindful of calorie, fat, and sodium content in these chips.

❖ Granola bars and trail mix are often marketed as healthy snacks and may be high in fiber or vitamins. Be aware that they often contain added sugar, fat, and sometimes trans fat.

❖ Avoid highly processed snacks which are high in sugar, sodium, and calories.

❖ Look for snacks that are pre-portioned to one serving size to help you be mindful of how much you are enjoying.

❖ Snacks are meant to hold you over until your next meal. The best way to accomplish this is by choosing snacks which are mainly high fiber carbohydrates and protein, not snacks loaded with sugar and fat.

❖ The best way to choose healthy snacks is to avoid the snack aisle all together and create your own healthy snacks at home.

*Check the next page for healthy snacks you can make yourself.*

# Snacks

## *Shopping Tips*

**Consider these healthy snacks:**

❖ Vegetables and hummus or homemade guacamole

❖ Fruit with natural, unsalted nut butter

❖ Non-fat Greek yogurt with fresh fruit

❖ Whole grain rice cake with natural, unsalted nut butter

❖ Part skim string cheese

❖ Fat-free pudding cup

❖ Frozen fruit such as mango or grapes

❖ Fruit with fat-free whipped topping

❖ Fresh fruit

❖ Homemade trail mix with nuts, whole grains, dried fruit, and a little bit of dark chocolate

❖ Air popped popcorn

❖ Fruit ice pops made with all natural fruit juices

❖ A hardboiled egg

❖ High fiber, low sugar cereal with fat-free milk

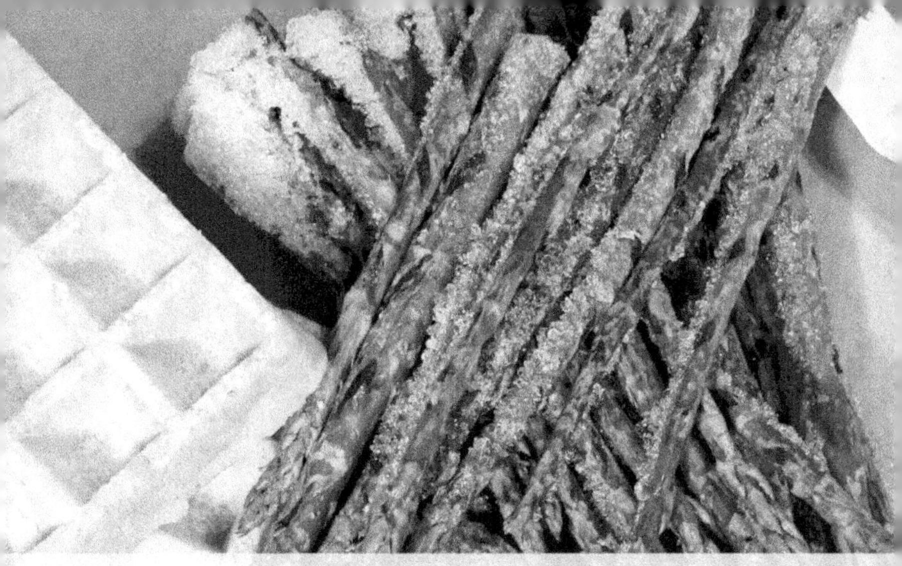

# Frozen
# Foods

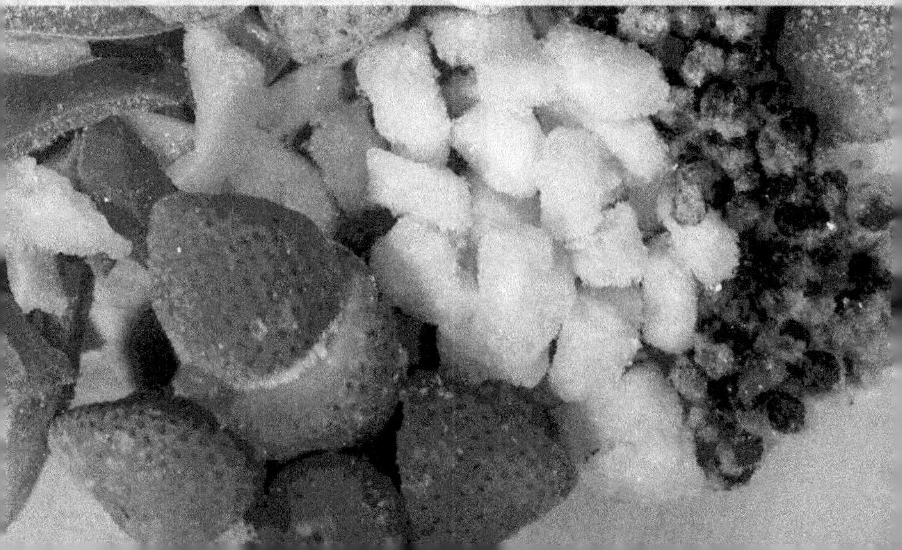

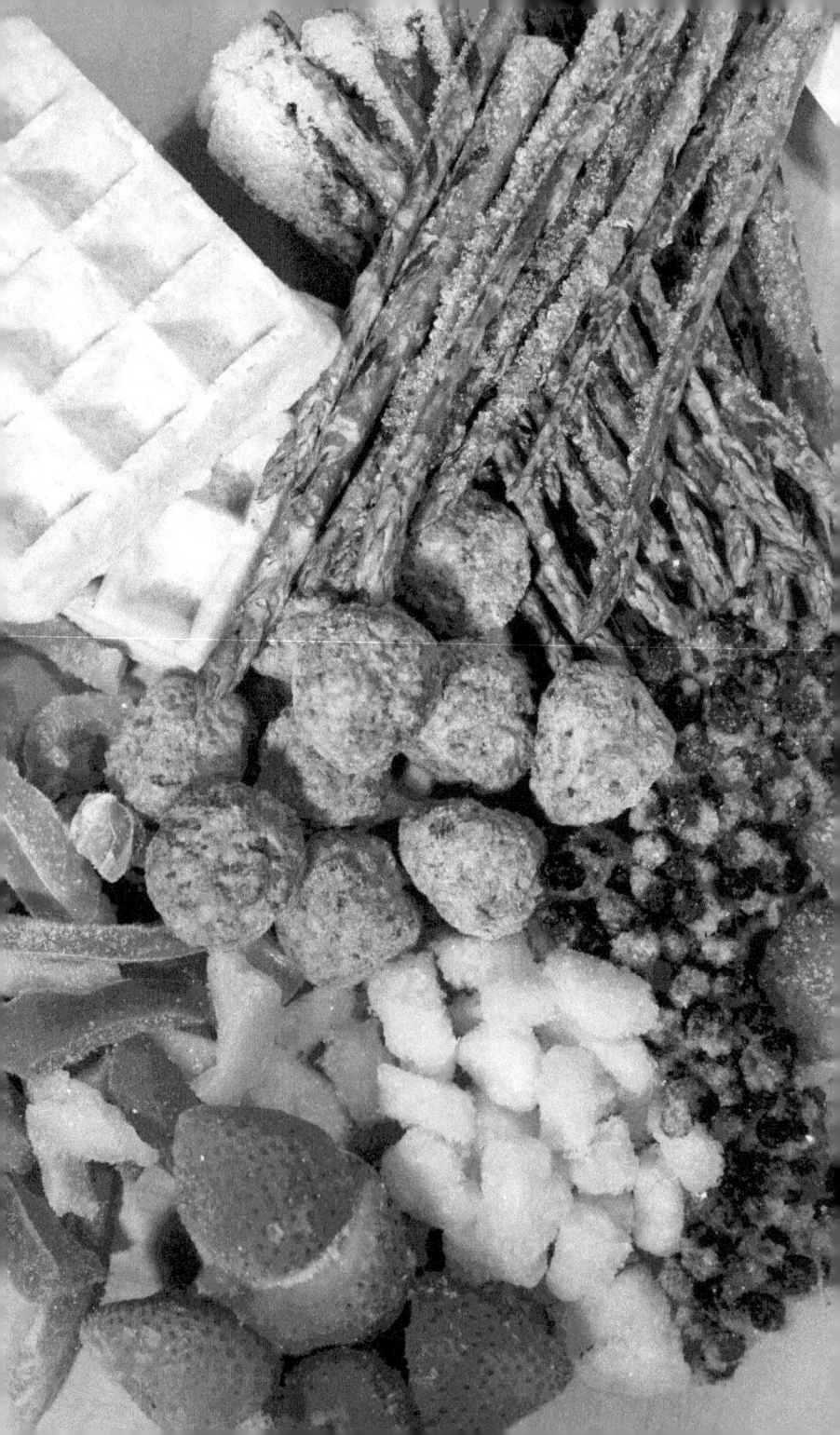

# Frozen Food

 Be aware of sodium, fat, and calorie content in frozen dishes. Many frozen meals contain far more sodium and calories than should be eaten in one meal.

**Frozen Meals**

❖ Look for "healthy", "lean", or "light" on packages. This is usually an indication that the item is more nutritious than others.

❖ Always check the label to ensure the item meets these general guidelines per meal:

› 500 or less calories.

› 3 grams or less saturated fat.

› 0 grams trans fat.

› 3 or more grams fiber.

› 600 milligrams or less sodium.

› No MSG (monosodium glutamate).

# Frozen Food

## *Navigating the Label*

 Be mindful of the sugar and calorie content of frozen desserts. Take note of serving size and be sure to mind your servings.

### Frozen Fruits & Vegetables

❖ The only ingredients should be fruits and vegetables with no added sugars, syrups, or sauces.

❖ Look for "flash frozen" on the package for fruits and vegetables that were picked and frozen at their peak ripeness.

❖ Choose plain vegetables or vegetable mixtures without cheese sauces or added fats such as butter.

❖ If you do choose vegetables that are prepared in a sauce, be aware of the calorie and sodium content.

### Desserts

❖ Look for desserts that are 150 calories or less per serving.

❖ Compare calories, sugar, and fat in frozen desserts.

❖ Choose low fat ice cream, sherbet, sorbet or frozen yogurt instead of premium ice cream.

# Frozen Food

## *Shopping Tips*

❖ When your favorite fruits and vegetables are out of season, try picking them up from the frozen aisle. They will be more available and more affordable.

❖ Check that fruits and vegetables have not frozen into a single clump. This means they have been thawed and refrozen which decreases the nutrient content.

❖ Frozen shrimp come in sizes ranging from small to jumbo. Check serving sizes for what you purchase.

❖ Whole grain waffles or bagels, lean breakfast meats, and egg substitutes in the freezer aisle make for a quick healthy breakfast.

❖ Avoid buying foods that are breaded and pre-fried by the manufacturer.

❖ For frozen meals that are 300 calories, add a cup of fresh vegetables, a salad or a fruit to add extra nutrition to the meal.

❖ Pass on tubs of ice cream that can cause you to overindulge. Instead, buy desserts that are already pre-portioned such as ice pops.

❖ If you have a blender, try making your own treat by blending frozen fruit and low fat milk for a healthier version of ice cream.

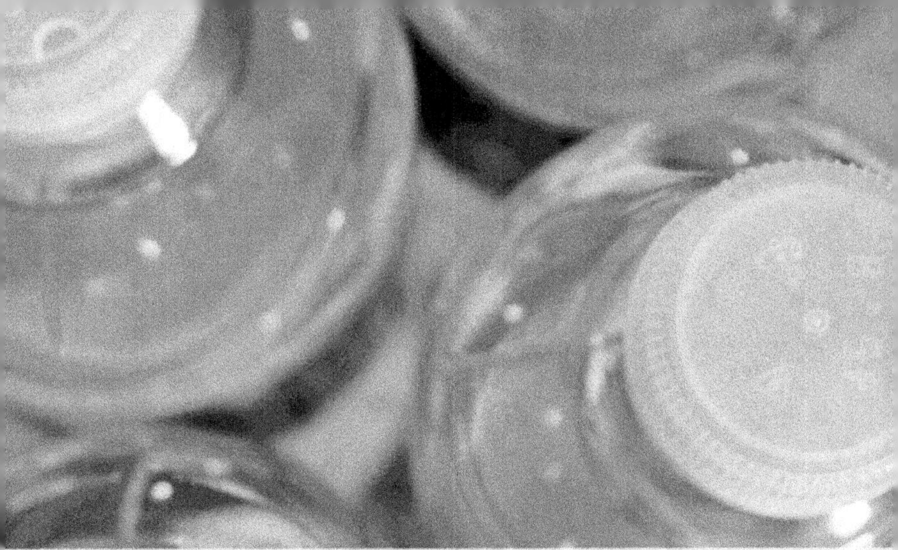

# Beverages

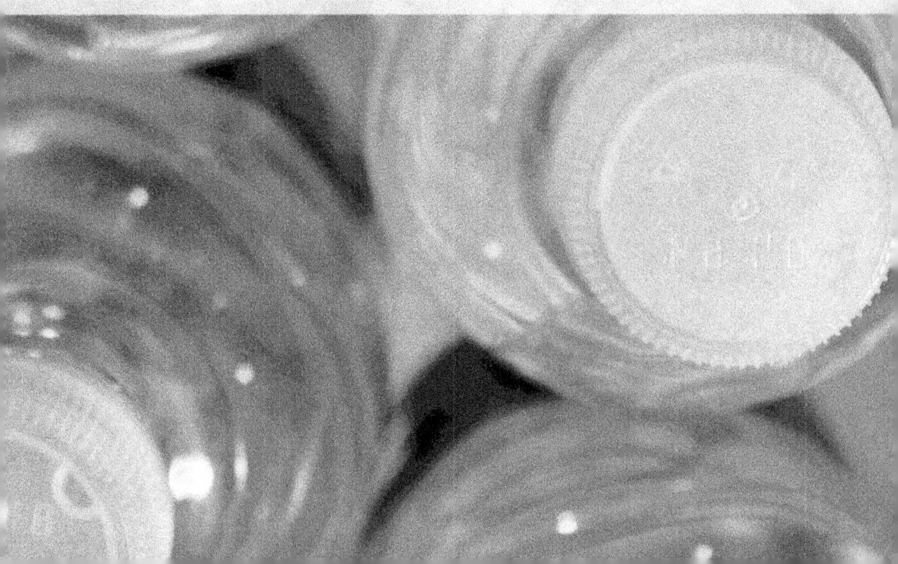

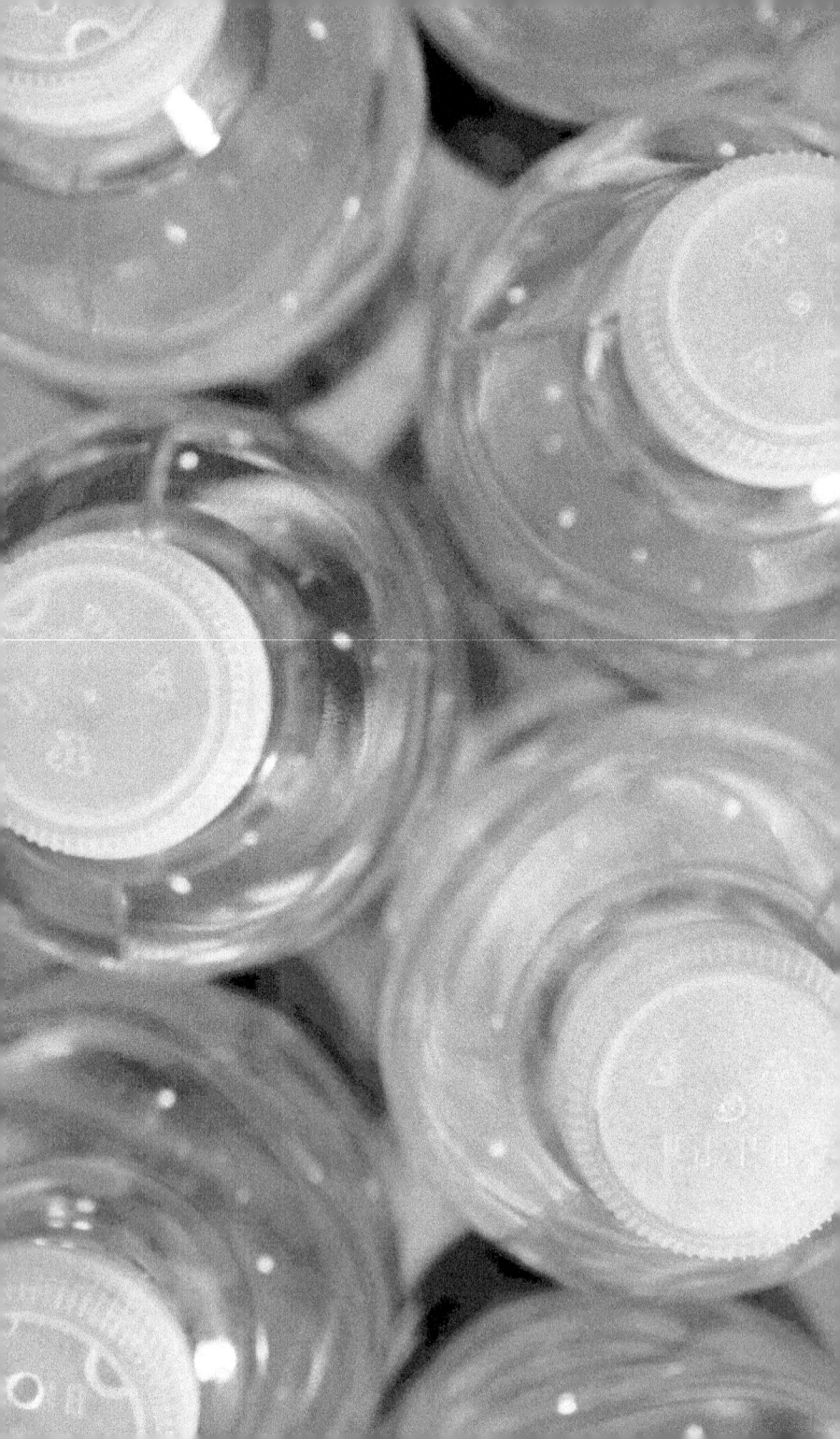

# Beverages

## *Navigating the Label*

 Sugar is the major culprit in many beverages that leads to weight gain.

Take note of serving sizes. One bottle often contains more than one serving.

❖ Look for "100% fruit juice" on fruit juice labels. Avoid artificial flavors, colors, and sweeteners.

❖ Juice cocktails, beverages, punches, or blends contain between 10-99% fruit juice and may contain added sweeteners or other ingredients that are not naturally found in fruit juice.

❖ "Fruit drinks" are flavored water which contains no actual fruit juice and therefore does not offer nutrients from fruit.

❖ "Diet" drinks may not contain as many calories or sugar but this is because they are made with chemicals and artificial sweeteners. They are not the healthiest options.

❖ Be aware of the high content of sugar, caffeine, and other stimulants and chemicals in energy drinks.

❖ "Sports drinks" tend to contain a lot of sugar. For a more nutritious post-workout drink, buy or make your own chocolate milk which contains natural sugars, carbohydrates, and nutrients.

# Beverages

 Alcohol is a major source of empty calories and can hinder your health goals.

❖ Water is your best beverage option and should be your go-to drink.

❖ Purchasing a washable, re-useable water bottle can save money usually spent on disposable bottles and will cut down on plastic waste.

❖ If you decide to drink alcohol, opt for light beer, dry wine, or liquor mixed with seltzer and a splash of juice for flavor.

❖ Instead of soda, try switching to seltzer or carbonated water. Add flavor with fresh fruits such as citrus fruits.

❖ Try apple cider rather than apple juice. It contains more fiber and antioxidants.

❖ If you enjoy juice but want to reduce the sugar and calorie content, fill just half your cup with juice and the other half with water

❖ Avoid any artificial colors, sweeteners, and high fructose corn syrup.

❖ Avoid using creamers and sugar which add calories. Use low-fat or fat-free milk instead.

# References

American Heart Association. (n.d.). *Try these tips for heart-healthy grocery shopping.* Retrieved from http://www.heart.org/HEARTORG/ GettingHealthy/NutritionCenter/HeartSmartShopping/Grocery-Shopping_UCM_

American Pregnancy Association. (2014.). *Mercury levels in fish.* Retrieved from http://americanpregnancy.org/pregnancyhealth/fishmercury.htm

Blonz, E. (2013). *How to Buy Dairy: Milk, yogurt, cheese.* Retrieved from http://www.berkeleywellness.com/healthy-eating/food/article/how-buy-dairy-milk-yogurt-cheese

Boar's Head. (n.d.). *Pile on the flavor, not the salt.* Retrieved from http://boarshead.com/health-wellness/information/lower-sodium/

Centers of Disease Control and Prevention. (2011).*Rethink your drink.* Retrieved from http://www.cdc.gov/healthyweight/healthy_eating/drinks.html

Center for Food Safety. (n.d.). *Soups, sauces & canned foods.* Retrieved from http://www.centerforfoodsafety.org/issues/311/ge-foods/non-gmo-shoppers-guide-325/1940/soups-sauces-and-canned-foods

Clemson University. (2014.). *Choosing breakfast cereals.* Retrieved from http://www.clemson.edu/extension/hgic/food/nutrition/food_shop_prep/food_shop/hgic4224.html

Dairy Council of California. (n.d.). *Types of milk.* Retrieved from http://www.healthyeating.org/Milk-Dairy/Dairy-Facts/Types-of-Milk.aspx

Environmental Working Group. (2015). Retrieved from http://www.ewg.org/foodnews/index.php

Foco, Z. (RD). (n.d.). *On-the-go: A guide to frozen meals.* Retrieved from http://www.diabetes.org/mfa-recipes/tips/2012-04/on.html

# References

Gold, M. V. (2007). *Organic production/organic food: information access tools*. Retrieved from http://www.nal.usda.gov/afsic/pubs/ofp/ofp.shtml

*Guide to buying frozen food*. (n.d.) Retrieved from http://www.realsimple.com/health/nutrition-diet/healthy-eating/guide-to-buying-frozen-food/view-all

Huffington Post. (2013). *The healthiest and unhealthiest salad dressings*. Retrieved from http://www.huffingtonpost.com/the-daily-meal/the-healthiest-and-unheal_b_3517759.html

Hand, B, (RD). (n.d.). *What to look for when buying bread*. Retrieved from http://www.womansday.com/health-fitness/diet-weight-loss/what-to-look-for-when-buying-bread-116101

Jaret, P. (n.d.). *Reading the ingredient label: What to look for*. Retrieved from http://www.webmd.com/food-recipes/features/healthy-ingredients

Ham, L. (n.d.) *About organic produce*. Retrieved from https://www.ocf.berkeley.edu/~lhom/organictext.html

Marcason, W. (2014). *Quick guide to food label terms*. Retrieved from http://www.eatright.org/resource/food/nutrition/nutrition-facts-and-food-labels/quick-guide-to-food-label-terms

Mayo Clinic Staff. (2014). *Health tip: Buy lean meat*. Retrieved from http://www.mayoclinic.org/healthy-living/nutrition-and-healthy-eating/in-depth/food-and-nutrition/art-20048095

Medicine Net. (n.d.). *Health tip: Buy lean meat*. Retrieved from http://www.medicinenet.com/script/main/art.asp?articlekey=156919

MedlinePlus, National Institutes of Health. (2014, 02 03). *Healthy grocery shopping*. Retrieved from http://www.nlm.nih.gov/medlineplus/ency/patientinstructions/000336.htm

# References

Minnesota Dept. of Health. (n.d.). *Fresh choices! changing for the better.* Retrieved from http://www.health.state.mn.us/divs/fh/wic/newwicfoods/ppt/faqs/milk.html

National Heart, Lung, and Blood Institute. (2014).*Low-calorie, lower fat alternative foods*. Retrieved from http://www.nhlbi.nih.gov/health/public/h1eart/obesity/lose_wt/lcal_fat.htm

New York Times ,Fitness and Nutrition. (n.d.). *Recipes for health: Quinoa.* Retrieved from http://topics.nytimes.com/top/news/health/series/recipes_for_health/quinoa/

*Safe Handling.* (n.a.). http://meatsafety.org/ht/d/sp/i/26023/pid/26023

Self Nutrition Data. (n.d.). *Beef, ground, 95% lean meat / 5% fat, patty, cooked, pan-broiled [hamburger]*. Retrieved from http://nutritiondata.self.com/facts/beef-products/6190/2

Stevenson, H. (2008). *The labeling system*. Retrieved from http://www.naturalnews.com/023711_fruit_labels_health.html

*The basics of the nutrition facts panel.* (2014). Retrieved from http://www.eatright.org/resource/food/nutrition/nutrition-facts-and-food-labels/the-basics-of-the-nutrition-facts-panel

*Understanding food marketing terms* (2014). Retrieved from http://www.eatright.org/resource/food/nutrition/nutrition-facts-and-food-labels/understanding-food-marketing-terms

United States Dept. Agriculture, A. (1995). *How to buy eggs*. Retrieved from http://www.ams.usda.gov/AMSv1.0/getfile?dDocName=STELDEV3022056

WebMD. (n.d.). *Nutty about peanut butter*. Retrieved from http://www.webmd.com/food-recipes/features/nutty-about-peanut-butter

www.ingramcontent.com/pod-product-compliance
Lightning Source LLC
Chambersburg PA
CBHW060434290526
45791CB00002B/946